RUNNER'S WORLD. THE
RUNNER'S BODY

RUNNER'S WORLD® THE

RUNNER'S BODY

How The Latest Exercise Science Can
Help You Run Stronger, Longer, and Faster

ROSS TUCKER, PhD, AND JONATHAN DUGAS, PhD
WITH MATT FITZGERALD

Rodale books may be purchased for business or promotional use or for special sales. For information, please write to: Special Markets Department, Rodale Inc., 733 Third Avenue, New York, NY 10017

Runner's World is a registered trademark of Rodale Inc.

Printed in the United States of America
Rodale Inc. makes every effort to use acid-free ♾, recycled paper ♻.

Illustrations by Sandy Freeman

Book design by Susan Eugster

Library of Congress Cataloging-in-Publication Data
Tucker, Ross.
   Runner's world, the runner's body : how the latest exercise science can help you run stronger, longer, and faster / by Ross Tucker and Jonathan Dugas ; with Matt Fitzgerald.
     p.   cm.
   Includes index.
   ISBN-13 978-1-60529-861-0 paperback
   1. Running—Physiological aspects.   2. Exercise—Physiological aspects.   3. Running—Training.
I. Dugas, Jonathan. II. Fitzgerald, Matt. III. Runner's world. IV. Title.
RC1220.R8T83 2009
613.7'172—dc22
                                                      2009008203

Distributed to the trade by Macmillan

2   4   6   8   10   9   7   5   3   1   paperback

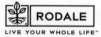

RODALE
LIVE YOUR WHOLE LIFE™

We inspire and enable people to improve their lives and the world around them

For more of our products visit **rodalestore.com** or call 800-848-4735

*This book is dedicated to
curious runners everywhere.*

[Contents]

[Acknowledgments]

Ross Tucker:

This book was inspired by a combination of too many people to name over too long a period to recall. However, special mentions go to Yumna, Sacha, George, Tami, Dale, Tertius, and Rob vd V. Thank you for your support, friendship, and encouragement. Rob B and Bruce Beckett provided questioning minds, ideas, and the support that turns "mere" science into the kind of content hopefully produced in this book. Thanks to the de Witt family for making their home available for a week and to Karlien for help with the content. For my grandmother, Joyce.

Jonathan Dugas

Thanks to my co-authors Matt and Ross for all their hard work throughout this process, especially Matt for your guidance and insight, and Ross for all your technical edits and thoughts. Special thanks to my loving wife Lara for her support during the writing of this book.

Matt Fitzgerald:

I would like to thank the following special individuals for their direct and indirect contributions to this rewarding project: Jason Ash, Courtney Conroy, Eric Cressey, John Duke, Gear Fisher, Nataki Fitzgerald, Michael Fredericson, Donavon Guyot, Jane Hahn, Brad Hudson, Asker Jeukendrup, Linda Konner, T.J. Murphy, and Tim Noakes.

[Introduction]

The human body is a marvel. Its 100 trillion frequently replaced cells (not to mention another one trillion foreign bacteria cells that live inside us) cooperate in an exquisitely choreographed dance of chemical, electrical, and magnetic interaction that is influenced in countless ways by the surrounding environment. The human body would be fascinating to study even if each of us did not inhabit one. But the fact that we *are* human bodies makes every new thing we learn about them an awe-inspiring step of self-discovery.

And each of these steps has the power to immediately change our lives. For example, when a person first learns that the human body requires regular exposure to natural sunlight to produce adequate amounts of vitamin D, she might make efforts to get outdoors more.

Considering that you have picked up this book, we expect that one of the ways in which you hope to change your life is by improving your running performance. Most major universities have exercise science departments where professionals like us conduct research that is relevant to the performance interests of athletes, including runners just like you. It is hardly necessary to hold a PhD in kinesiology to improve as a runner, but gaining a better understanding of the physiological underpinnings of running performance will certainly give you the wherewithal to make helpful changes to your training, with fewer missteps.

More important than remembering every detail about the physiology of running is understanding the basic principles that underlie those details. The details change as science progresses, but the principles do not. You can always fall back on the principles to guide your decision making as a runner. None of this book's details is as important as the single most fundamental tenet of exercise physiology. If you come away from this book having learned only one thing, we hope that it is a full appreciation of this vital principle: the principle of stress and adaptation. Understanding it is almost like having a coach to guide you through every step of your journey as a runner.

Stress and Adaptation

To understand the processes that occur in your body when you train, it helps to go back to 1936 and the work of a medical doctor named Hans Selye, who is regarded as the first person to demonstrate the existence of the so-called stress response. His work involved exposing mice to various "stressors," including cold environments, surgical injury, doses of diverse drugs, extracts of other foreign tissues, and even excessive exercise (yes, running and other forms of exercise can be stressors!), and then measuring the physiological responses to each one. Selye found that regardless of the initial source of stress, the mice reacted with a very typical pattern of responses: an initial *alarm* stage, followed by a period of *resistance or adaptation*, when the organism gets stronger and performs better (which is, of course, where you want to be as a runner). This leads, if the stress is not removed, to *exhaustion*.

A greater understanding of the physiology of running can help you get into, and remain in, that stage of adaptation and avoid the unwanted stage of exhaustion, in which your body fails to adapt and instead falls prey to overtraining, injury, and burnout.

THE EARLY PHASE: ALARM BELLS RINGING

Running stresses the body—just ask your nonrunning friends how they would feel if they accompanied you on tomorrow's training run! In the initial, alarm stage, when that stress is first applied, your body can change in one of three ways, depending on the magnitude of the stress:

1. If the training stimulus is of optimal duration and intensity (you'll see exactly what we mean by "optimal" later on), your body begins adapting.

2. If the training stress is too hard, you will break down almost immediately, develop injuries, feel excessive fatigue, and fail to recover from one day to the next. All in all, training will be a very unpleasant experience, and you will probably retire from running or take up another sport.

3. If the training stimulus is relatively weak and does not really test your physiological systems, your body will not see any need to make adaptations, and you will remain at the same level. This is a concern for runners who have reached a performance plateau. You might have been training for

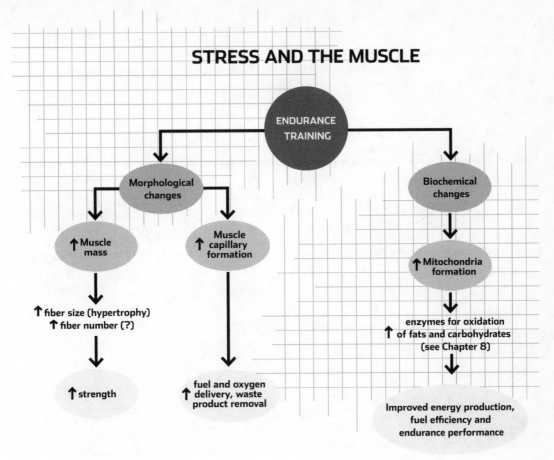

STRESS AND THE MUSCLE

Selye's General Adaptation Principle

months or years and find that you're no longer improving. One possible reason (there are a few) is insufficient training stress.

So it's absolutely vital that you manage training stress wisely by controlling the various elements that determine its magnitude.

These elements include:

→ **Volume,** which is made up of two aspects:

- **Duration:** How far or for how long you run
- **Frequency:** How often you run

→ **Intensity:** How hard you run.

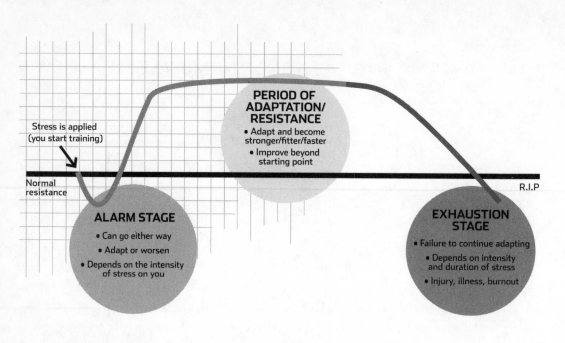

Stress is applied
(you start training)

Normal
resistance

R.I.P

PERIOD OF ADAPTATION/ RESISTANCE
- Adapt and become stronger/fitter/faster
- Improve beyond starting point

ALARM STAGE
- Can go either way
- Adapt or worsen
- Depends on the intensity of stress on you

EXHAUSTION STAGE
- Failure to continue adapting
- Depends on intensity and duration of stress
- Injury, illness, burnout

Period of adaptation resistance

This is often the straw that breaks the camel's back, since it's subjective and therefore difficult to measure and control.

→ **Recovery:** How much time you take off between hard training efforts. Also known as *rest* (which can be *active* or *complete*), recovery is the most important component, and there are different types:

- **Recovery within days** (when you break up a run with periods of walking or slower running, for example)
- **Recovery between days**
- **Recovery between weeks and months.** All must be managed wisely to make the most of your training.

The interaction of these components determines how your body adapts. If either the volume or the intensity is excessive, your body may never adapt or move beyond the alarm stage. Instead, it may slide off into injury and exhaustion. This is an almost universal experience among runners, most of whom will, at some point, take on too much too soon or for too long, and become injured. This most often happens to novice runners, whose enthusiasm we cannot fault as they dive passionately into a new activity they enjoy. Fortunately, the body will eventually recover, allowing another shot at training, hopefully the right way.

However, even when the stress is correctly managed, the body's adaptation can be a difficult experience—stiff muscles and fatigue are common in the first week or two of any training program and whenever volume or intensity is increased. Runners are constantly walking a tightrope between adaptation and physiological failure. As a runner, it's important to understand how to be cautious enough to avoid injury, while at the same time being aggressive enough to stimulate adaptation.

A PERIOD OF ADAPTATION: STRONGER, FASTER, FITTER

If you manage the stress carefully, your body will move into the stage of adaptation, in which you become a better runner. This is the remarkable result of an innumerable amount of physiological responses, most of which you'll never even be aware. These responses include adaptations in your muscles, nerves, bones, heart, lungs, brain, and all the other tissues in your body. You become better at taking in oxygen and then extracting it from your lungs before pumping it to your muscles, thanks to your stronger heart and more numerous blood vessels. You also improve your ability to use carbohydrates and fats to generate the energy you need to power muscle contraction. Your brain responds to training by allowing you to run ever closer to your physiological limit, which itself moves higher, thanks to the metabolic and muscular changes induced by training. In the pages that follow, we'll look at what allows some runners to make these adaptations far more effectively than the average person, running faster and farther than most of us ever will. We can learn from their gifts, and by understanding the physiology of performance, we can borrow training techniques that will allow us to move closer to the level of those elite runners.

An additional aspect of the stress response is that the adaptations you make will be specific to that particular stress; this is called the Law of Specificity. For example, longer, slower running will improve your endurance, while track workouts and interval sessions will increase your speed. The marriage of all these different aspects is what produces the package that turns you into a faster runner. When you get your training right, you will recognize that your running is becoming easier, faster, and more enjoyable. Our aim in this book is to explain the physical adaptations underlying this process and how you can target and make the most of them with strategies that maximize the time you spend in the period of adaptation.

THE STAGE OF EXHAUSTION: TOO MUCH OF A GOOD THING

If the stress of training is too intense or lasts too long, your body cannot adapt. Instead, it deteriorates until you reach the stage of exhaustion. It is in this stage that you become injured, burned out, and overtrained. Running is no longer pleasant, and your performances steadily decline, despite your most diligent efforts. Your reaction to your declining performance may be to train harder still, which only accelerates your downward spiral. You might get sick often, missing weeks of training at a time. We'll offer strategies that will help you avoid entering this stage.

The key to avoiding exhaustion is *change management:* You have to carefully manage the initial stress, the recovery, and the adaptation. Even experienced runners, with thousands of training miles behind them, must be aware of the constant need to manage change. For example, a week off represents change, so the return to running must be managed. The start of a new phase of training, perhaps with more speedwork, requires the same focus.

Your Running Body

Imagine taking a guided tour through your own body as it runs, recovers, and adapts to running. There does not yet exist a camera small or mobile enough to lead such a tour, but this book is the next best thing. It divides the body into five distinct functional systems—musculoskeletal, cardiorespiratory, metabolic, nervous, and immune—and devotes a section to each. Within each part, individual chapters address specific topics that will help you optimize each system's contribution to your running performance.

Part 1 looks at your muscles, bones, and joints. You will learn what causes postrun muscle soreness and how to reduce its negative effects on your training. You'll also discover the causes of the most common running injuries, how to prevent and overcome them, and much more.

Part 2 is all about your cardiorespiratory system, addressing topics such as what makes some runners more efficient than others and how you can become more efficient. We'll also debunk the many myths about hydration and running.

The metabolic system is the subject of Part 3; you'll come away from it with a better understanding of how to fuel your body for maximum performance by using a science-based strategy to achieve your optimal running weight, plus other practical lessons. We'll move on to the nervous system in Part 4, with chapters on the role of the brain in fatigue and technique, and the effects of running on brain health and mental well-being.

In fact, we'll name one of those brain benefits right here: Running actually makes you smarter. But it also works the other way around. The smarter you are about your running, the better you run. We're confident that after completing this guided tour through your runner's body, you will be a smarter, healthier, and more efficient runner than ever before.

PART 1

The Musculo

skeletal System

Becoming the best runner you can be requires a basic understanding of human anatomy. Just as an engineer must know precisely what parts go into a machine to make it work, we have to build up our understanding of what goes into your body. So bear with us as we lay out this simple hierarchy of organization in the body, beginning with the smallest piece, the cell, and ending with the complete organism, you.

The most basic unit of the body, the cell, is a stand-alone object that performs a specific task depending on its type—skin cell, muscle cell, bone cell. As small as it is, however, a cell has even smaller things inside it. Called organelles, these carry out specialized functions that come together to help the cell perform its job—think of different parts of a car assembly plant, for example.

When similar cells get together, they form tissue, and organized tissue forms an organ. Within an organ, cells and tissues act as functional units that perform a very specific job—for example, producing tension to help pump blood in the heart. And therein lies the purpose of an organ: to perform a large task within the body, such as the heart's labor of pumping blood throughout the body to all the other cells and tissues.

Two or more organs or tissues that work together to achieve an even bigger task form a system. The musculoskeletal system is the collection of muscle and bone tissues that work together to produce movement. Finally, all the systems in the body work together to keep you, the runner, alive and running.

This musculoskeletal system in itself comprises two individual systems, the neuromuscular system and the skeletal system. The neuromuscular system initiates movement, with your muscles contracting or relaxing in response to signals that travel from the brain via the spinal cord. However, muscle contractions by themselves cannot produce movement. It is the skeletal system that translates muscle tension into movement. Each muscle is attached to two or more bones that form lever arms across our joints. This is the mechanical arrangement that allows us to make the type of movements that allow us to run.

The musculoskeletal system produces the movement that allows us to run. Human movement is incredibly complex, and even "simple" movements are achieved through a series of neural, chemical, and physical steps.

Chapter 1

Meat Machines

With the majority of our mass made up of skeletal muscle, we are indeed meat machines. The body of the typical male runner is approximately 15 to 20 percent body fat; that of his female counterpart is roughly 10 to 15 percent higher. This leaves the remaining 80 to 85 percent (for a male) lean mass. Part of that mass is bone and other organs, but muscle comprises the biggest portion by far. More important, our muscles and skeleton allow us to perform many complex movements, such as running.

Your musculoskeletal system is truly the foundation of your running, and your running can only be as good as your foundation is healthy and balanced. In this chapter, we will explain first how your body is structured and how muscle actually works. Then we'll describe some common irregularities in this system and show you some simple ways to correct them.

A Tug-of-War and a Power Stroke

To understand how muscles actually contract to move our limbs, let's begin with the example of the quadriceps, the group of four muscles on the front of the thigh that is one of the primary muscle groups involved in running. The illustration on page 12 depicts the quadriceps at the point where it attaches to a tendon. It is shown in cross section so that you can see the increasingly smaller parts, all the way down to the very smallest unit: a single *myofibril*, which is even smaller than the muscle cell itself and contains the two essential components that actually produce movement.

These two parts are called *actin* and *myosin*. These two "filaments" work together to cause the muscle to contract, or shorten, thereby producing muscle movement. To understand this process better, let's use the analogy of a team of people (myosin) pulling a rope (actin). Attached to the other end of the rope is an object they want to pull toward them. An important point is that team members cannot hold the rope at just any position—there are specific sites or "handles" that they must grasp. The people can get hold of these positions only when the coach (the brain) makes them available. The brain sends a nerve impulse that opens tiny channels in a part of the muscle called the *sarcoplasmic reticulum*. These channels release calcium, which engages in a biochemical process to expose the actin handles to which myosin can bind. Once this has happened, the team grabs hold and is ready to pull. Every single pull is a highly energized reaction known as a *power stroke*, which shortens the muscle a tiny bit using energy from a molecule called *ATP*, the fundamental energy for all muscle work. After each power stroke, each team member must release the rope to allow the muscle to lengthen again. This step requires additional ATP, because the team members have just used all their energy to perform the first power stroke. As another molecule of ATP bonds to the myosin, they release the actin and get ready to grab (bind) once again to shorten the muscle

a bit more. This series of events repeats until you have completed the movement—for example, contracting your quadriceps during the footstrike phase of running. (Note that if additional ATP is not available, the team members cannot release the rope, and the muscle is unable to relax. This is the explanation for the postmortem condition known as rigor mortis: The body can no longer produce energy; as a result, all the team members remain attached to the rope. The muscle fails to relax, instead becoming stiff and immobile.)

The really amazing thing about muscle contraction is that these microscopic actions happen repeatedly and very quickly—hundreds of times in the second or two it takes you to flex your hips and knees to sit down and read this book. It takes literally milliseconds to complete them, so it's easy to see why a complex movement such as running is truly an incredible physiological and biochemical feat. And perhaps more impressive is that we are not even conscious of what is happening inside our muscles as we move.

Lending Support: The Bones

Of course, to produce movement, each end of a muscle must be attached to a bone, and the muscle and bones must be arranged in such a way as to form a joint. But before we talk about the structure and function of joints, let's sort out bone tissue and the skeletal system. As runners, we are most interested in the *long bones*, the ones in our legs and arms. Each of the long bones has a lengthy middle section called a shaft, inside of which is the bone marrow.

Most of us probably think of bones as quite dry, dead things. In fact, bone is a living tissue much like the rest of the body. The primary purposes of the bones and skeleton are to provide support and structure for the body and to allow movement by attaching to muscle. But in addition, bones also store and then release calcium and phosphorus when required by the body; the bones of the rib cage specifically protect the vital organs in the chest; and bone marrow produces blood cells. Bone is also a tissue that is broken down and regenerated on an ongoing basis and can be made weaker or stronger in much the same way as the muscles can. So the skeleton is very much alive and active.

Like any other organ or system in the body, bone becomes stronger when it is stressed regularly, and it deteriorates when it is not used enough. In this case, "stressed" means loaded through impact and tension, as occurs during running. For the best illustration of this, look at astronauts. Their bones are unloaded and underutilized during lengthy stays in the zero-gravity environment of space. When they arrive back on Earth, their bones are often so weak that they can barely support the astronaut's body weight. At the other extreme are individuals who train excessively, loading their bones tens of thousands of times every day without ever allowing time for recovery and adaptation. This is a surefire way to become injured, and we often see overload in athletes with bone stress injuries, which we'll cover in more detail in Chapter 4.

The good news is that just walking around and carrying your weight provides sufficient loading to ensure a healthy skeleton. Even better, a proper running program that correctly manages training stress will result in stronger bones. Running is a great way to promote healthy bones. As a runner, you can cheat the aging process. Between the ages of about 25 and 30 years, your body stops laying down more bone. At this stage, a weight-bearing sport like running (along with ingesting sufficient calories and calcium) will actually reduce the rate at which your bones weaken and the rate at which you lose bone mass. That's why being active while you're young is so vital—you get yourself into the best possible position before the inevitable decline happens. Being a lifelong runner who remains healthy while properly managing training over the long run (literally and metaphorically) lowers your risk of the two major bone diseases, osteopenia and osteoporosis, which we'll discuss in more detail in Chapter 3.

Providing More Structure Still: The Joints

Muscles produce tension on bones, and bones provide support and protection. The missing piece of the movement puzzle is the point at which two bones meet: the joint. The musculoskeletal system can be effectively described as a series of levers, with each lever having three specific components:

1. Load: This is the force against which you must move the lever. If you hold this book in your hand and curl your biceps, the book is the load you are moving.

2. Effort: This is the force you must apply to make the lever move. In the biceps example, effort is the force exerted by your muscle in an attempt to elevate this book in your hand. Note that the effort is not necessarily always up to the task of causing movement—if the load is exactly equal to the effort, then the book stays in the same place. If the load is greater, then the book won't move. Only when the effort is greater than the load can you produce movement.

3. Fulcrum: This is the point around which the lever rotates. In your body, it is always a joint; in the biceps example, the fulcrum is your elbow.

The three parts of the musculoskeletal system—the muscles, bones, and joints—work together: The muscles provide the force, or effort; the bones act as lever arms; and the joints are the fulcrums about which our limb segments rotate. Thanks to their mutual cooperation, we can do everything from eating to running.

Ch-Ch-Changes

Now that you can appreciate the elegant and complex arrangement of the musculoskeletal system, we can delve into exactly what happens to that system when we stress it enough with running so that it makes adaptations. The chart on page 4 summarizes the way the body adapts to running.

In the Introduction, we first explained Selye's General Adaptation Principle. We described the body's general, nonspecific response to stressors, which occurs no matter what type of endurance activity you perform. For example, whether you take up running or rowing, adaptations such as increased blood volume and a decrease in resting heart rate take place. However, specific adaptations differ in magnitude and type, depending on the training stress that causes them. As a basic example, endurance running increases the density of mitochondria in the muscle cells, but *only in the legs*, not in the arms. Rowing, on the other hand, causes the same adaptations to happen in both arm and leg muscles. Sprint training causes a very different set of adaptations than endurance training. We'll cover some of these as we look at the structural (also called morphological) and biochemical changes that take place in muscle in response to running.

MORPHOLOGICAL METAMORPHOSES

When you either begin or progressively increase your running routine, the first major adaptation you might notice is that your leg musculature gets bigger. There are two ways a muscle can increase its size. Theoretically, the number of muscle fibers can increase, but there is scant evidence to suggest that this actually happens in humans. On the other hand, the size of each fiber can increase while the number of fibers remains constant. This is the effect you will see when you intensify training.

Another running-induced adaptation is one that we cannot see: the growth of more capillaries around the muscle. Capillaries are the microscopic blood vessels where nutrients, oxygen, and waste products such as carbon dioxide transfer between tissues and blood vessels. So why the extra pipes? Muscle is the body's most metabolically active tissue, especially during running. It demands a high rate of oxygen delivery so that it can produce ATP by burning fuels such as carbohydrates. Increasing the number of capillaries compares to building more roads to handle heavier traffic. This adaptation facilitates increased oxygen delivery to power muscle contractions and also allows the body to get rid of more waste products.

METABOLIC ADAPTATIONS

For much the same reason that capillary density increases, mitochondria in the muscle tissue increase as well. The mitochondria are the "engines" of the muscle, adding oxygen to fuels such as carbohydrates and fats while harnessing the energy from chemical reactions that ultimately produce ATP. Higher mitochondrial boosts the "horsepower" of the muscle, allowing us to produce more energy and run longer and faster.

The Law of Specificity applies: The type of training you do determines what kind of metabolic adaptations are produced. If you do a great deal of high-intensity running, such as sprint training and shorter interval sessions, your muscles respond by making more of the enzymes and chemicals that help you function during high-intensity running: You get better at producing ATP rapidly and buffering the hydrogen ions that are formed when you sprint. With distance training, you improve the efficiency of energy production, increasing mitochondria and all the enzymes they contain to help you produce more ATP for longer periods.

There is another benefit to this energy efficiency. As we will discuss more in Chapter 8, additional mitochondria provide your muscles greater capacity to use fat as a source of fuel. So as you become better and better trained, you will rely less on blood glucose and more on fat for running fuel. As a result, you'll finish a given run with higher concentrations of muscle and liver glycogen, which

Changing Your Equipment? Switching Fiber Types

You've probably read all about how distance runners have more Type I, or "slow twitch," muscle fibers, whereas sprinters have more Type II, or "fast twitch," fibers. One of the big debates still raging in exercise science is whether or not dedicated distance training over many years will change Type II fibers so that they either become Type I fibers or behave more like Type I fibers. Some scientists have produced data that they feel demonstrates such changes, but there is insufficient evidence to prove this conclusively.

will protect you from the dreaded bonk (hypoglycemia) that occurs when the liver's glycogen supply gets too low.

The really interesting thing about this change is that it cannot be explained entirely by the increase in mitochondrial density. The other mechanism at work is a change in the way you activate your muscles. This might mean that you are activating more or less muscle, depending on whether you are cruising during a two-hour run or doing a session of mile repeats. You may also be storing more triglycerides in the muscle, allowing you to more rapidly access fat as a fuel.

No matter what the cause of this change in fuel usage, the shift to fat as fuel will greatly enhance your endurance running performance.

Lactate, so long blamed for fatigue during exercise, is actually a product of carbohydrate metabolism. It is formed all the time, but at a much higher rate when you run faster—at that point, it starts to accumulate in the muscle and blood. When this happens, there is a range of other metabolic consequences. Some muscular adaptations to training will enhance your ability to take lactate out of the cytoplasm and into the muscle, where it can be burned as fuel. This is because exercise training increases the activity of a transporter that moves lactate into the mitochondria, where it can be used as fuel.

A Balancing Act

Today the average office worker spends almost nine and a half hours each weekday sitting (at the office, in the car going to and from the office, at home in front of the TV, and so forth). One consequence of such idleness is muscle and postural imbalances: Some muscles become abnormally tight, and others become very weak. Since your musculoskeletal system is the foundation of your running, any imbalances might have adverse effects on your body, in the form of injury or pain.

On the other hand, during running itself you use certain muscles all the time (e.g., your quads, hamstrings, glutes, and calves) and others much less often (i.e., those in your upper body). This, too, often creates a postural imbalance, and the consequences include pain and dysfunction in the lower back, knees, and other areas, and, as a result, reduced running performance.

Muscles are described as pairs of *agonists* and *antagonists*. A muscle or group of muscles that shorten and move a joint act as agonists. The muscle or group of muscles on the opposite side of the joint that relax to allow this movement act as antagonists. When the joint is moved in the opposite direction, the roles switch: The agonist becomes the antagonist and vice versa. While in the swing phase of running, for example, when you rapidly extend your knee in readiness for the next footstrike, your quads (agonist) extend your knee as your hamstrings (antagonist) slow down the joint and make sure your foot is in the right place to hit the ground when it needs to.

There are no rigorous definitions of muscle balance and imbalance. Rather, an imbalance is inferred when an injury or functional issue can be corrected by strengthening the muscles on one side of the affected joint and/or lengthening the muscles on the opposite side. Imbalances develop when you spend all your time running in a mostly straight line on the road, which is great for your quads and calves but leaves hip rotators like your glutes or core stabilizers a bit bored and understressed. As a result, the latter weaken while the others strengthen. Let's take a closer look at running-specific imbalances and their potential consequences.

LOWER LEGS

Strength and conditioning guru Michael Boyle has postulated that each major joint of the human body is designed primarily for either mobility or stability; the primary function alternates from joint to contiguous joint from the bottom to the top of the kinetic chain. The first major joint at the bottom of the chain is the ankle, and it is designed primarily for mobility. However, in most people today, the ankle joint lacks adequate mobility—specifically, its ability to dorsiflex (bring the toes up) is compromised.

Stiff ankles absorb less ground impact force and pass more force to the knees, increasing the risk of injury to the knees and other joints higher up the kinetic chain.

UPPER LEGS

Because many of us spend the better part of our days in a seated position, imbalances can develop between the quads and the hamstrings. While we sit, the hamstrings are flexed and the quads are stretched. This can lead to tight hamstrings and weak quads, a combination in runners that is commonly associated with knee pain.

HIPS AND PELVIS

The outer gluteal muscle, the gluteus medius, is a hip external rotator, and it can become weakened from the repetitive nature of road running. Any imbalance here renders the muscle less able to properly stabilize the hips and pelvis during running. Weakness in the hip abductors, on the outside of the thigh, is widespread in modern society, as well. Weak hip stabilizers are a major risk factor for the two most common running injuries: patellofemoral pain and iliotibial band syndrome.

SPINE AND SHOULDERS

For runners, a lack of cross-training or weight training targeting the upper body will lead to problems. Upper-body muscles are only mini-mally activated during running, so over many months and years, they will weaken to the point that they are barely able to do their jobs. The lumbar spine (lower back) and cervical spine (upper back) provide stability, while thoracic spine (midback) injuries tend to occur when you push the envelope a bit too far. When you go for your long run on Sunday morning after gardening all day Saturday, these fatigued muscles end up giving out before you finish your run. This forces other muscles, such as the psoas, which connects the lumbar spine to the upper thigh, to completely take over the job of stabilizing the lower back. The trouble with this is that these muscles really weren't designed for the job. Your psoas is normally a pretty powerful hip flexor. But if it has to both create stability at the lumbar spine *and* flex your hip, you experience compromised performance and increased risk of injuries such as hip flexor tendinitis.

Training for Body Balance

There is a variety of mobility and strengthening exercises you can do to put your muscles and joints back into their proper balance and thereby improve your running performance. Here is a selection of them—one for each part of the kinetic chain. Perform these exercises at least twice a week as part of your normal running program. The last three exercises—thoracic spine rotation, scapular pushup, and cable external shoulder rotation—are not running-specific, but we recommend them for building overall strength and fitness.

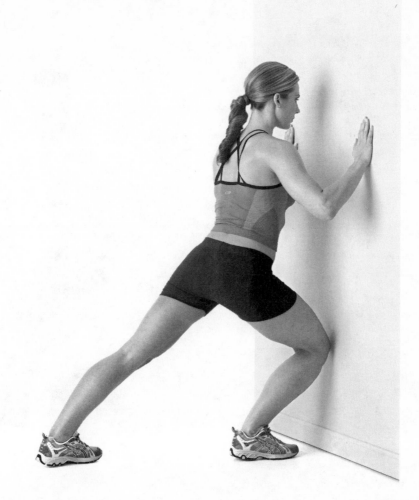

Ankle Mobilization

→INCREASES THE ANKLE JOINT'S ABILITY TO DORSIFLEX

Stand facing a wall, with the toes of one foot against it, and bend that knee to tap the wall. The opposite leg should extend slightly behind the working leg. Then slide your foot back a bit so that your toes are about an inch away from the wall, and again bend your knee to touch the wall. Keep moving back little by little until you get to the exact point where the kneecap is *barely* touching the wall. Make sure that your knee faces straight forward and not inward (knock-kneed) and that your heel remains on the floor the entire time. Perform 8 repetitions with each leg.

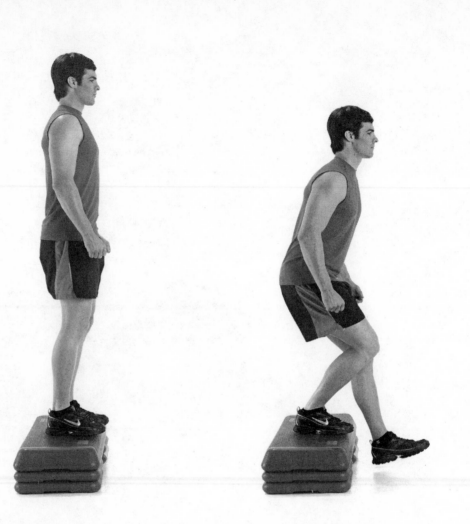

VMO Dip
→**STRENGTHENS THE VASTUS MEDIALIS TO IMPROVE KNEE STABILITY**

Stand on an exercise step that's 8 to 12 inches high. Pick up your left foot and slowly lower it toward the floor in front of the step by bending your right knee. Allow your left heel to touch the floor, but don't put any weight on it. Return to the starting position. Complete 8 to 12 repetitions and then switch legs.

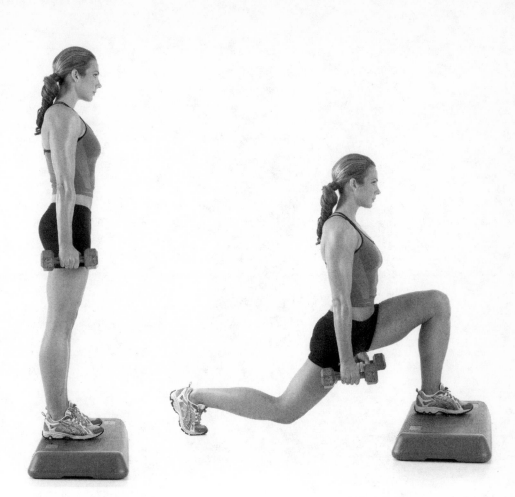

Elevated Backward Lunge
→**INCREASES MOBILITY OF THE HIPS**

Stand on a 4- to 6-inch step with your arms resting at your sides and a dumbbell in each hand.

Take a big step backward with one leg and bend both knees until the knee of the back leg grazes the floor, then thrust powerfully upward and forward off the rear foot to return to the starting position. Maintain an upright torso posture throughout the movement. Complete 10 reps with one leg, rest, and then switch legs.

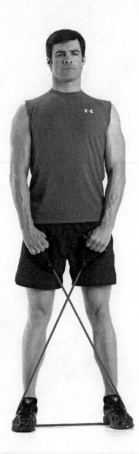

X-Band Walk
→STRENGTHENS THE HIP STABILIZERS

Loop a ½-inch- or 1-inch-thick exercise band under both feet and stand on top of it, with your feet roughly 12 inches apart. Cross the ends of the band to form an X and grasp one end in each hand. Pull your chest up and shoulders back and keep tension on the band throughout.

Start walking sideways with small lateral steps. (The leg toward the direction you're moving will have to overcome the band's tension for each step.) Keep your hips and shoulders level, and don't deviate forward or backward as you move to the side. When you perform this exercise correctly, you'll feel it in your glutes. Complete 10 steps in one direction and then 10 more in the opposite direction.

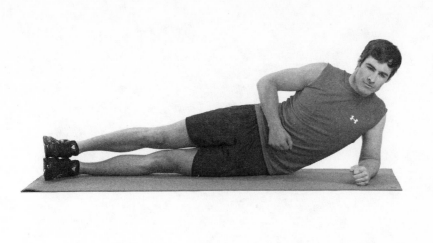

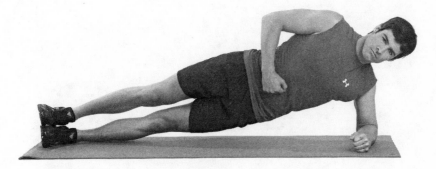

Side Bridge
→**STRENGTHENS THE LUMBAR SPINE STABILIZERS**

Lie on your right side with your legs fully extended and stacked and your right arm bent 90 degrees, with your forearm on the floor. Lift your hips until your body forms a straight line from neck to ankles. You may want to do this exercise in front of a mirror to make sure your hips don't sag toward the floor. Hold the bridge position for 20 to 30 seconds, and then flip over and repeat on the other side.

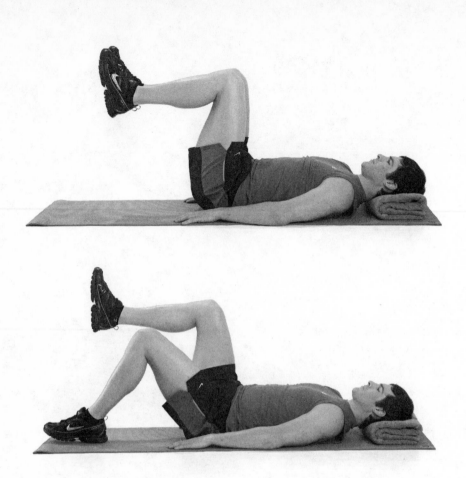

Lying Draw-In with Hip Flexion
→STRENGTHENS THE DEEP ABDOMINAL MUSCLES TO IMPROVE LUMBAR SPINE AND PELVIC STABILITY

Lie faceup, with your head supported by a large pillow or foam roller. Bend your knees 90 degrees and lift them so your thighs are perpendicular to the floor, feet together. Engage your deep abs by drawing your navel toward your spine and trying to flatten your lower back against the floor.

While holding this contraction, slowly lower your right foot to the floor. Immediately return to the starting position, then lower your left foot. If you find this movement easy, reengage the contraction in your deep abs. Lower each foot to the floor 8 to 10 times.

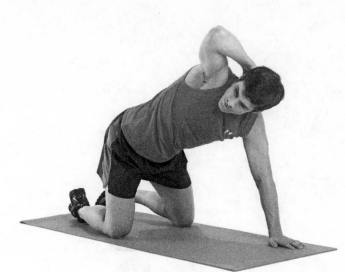

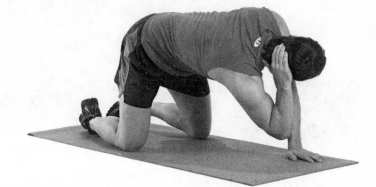

Thoracic Spine Rotation
→INCREASES MOBILITY OF THE THORACIC SPINE

Position yourself on all fours. Place your right hand on the back of your head.

Twist your torso to the left so that your right elbow swivels toward your left arm, which should be kept straight. Then rotate back, just past the starting position, so that your gaze is directed toward the wall to your right. Complete 12 rotations. Reverse arm positions and rotate in the opposite direction.

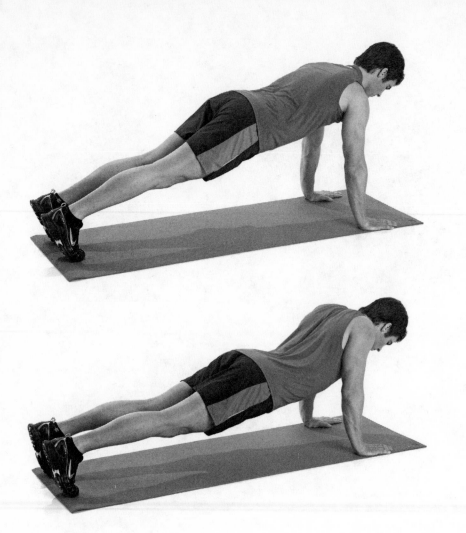

Scapular Pushup
→STRENGTHENS THE SCAPULAR STABILIZERS

Assume a standard pushup position. Keeping your elbows locked, retract your shoulder blades so that your torso sinks a couple of inches toward the floor. Now protract your shoulder blades fully, so that your upper back rounds slightly. Return to the starting position. Complete 12 to 15 repetitions.

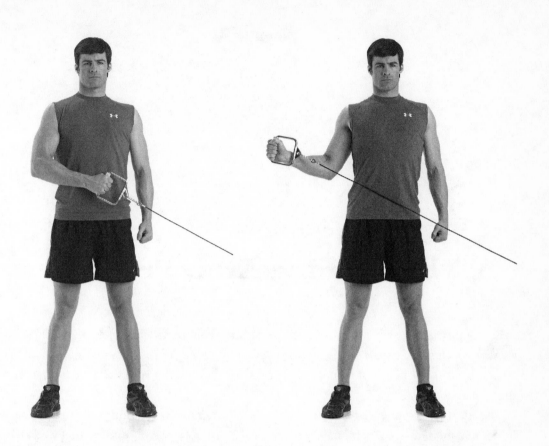

Cable External Shoulder Rotation

→STRENGTHENS THE ROTATOR CUFF MUSCULATURE TO IMPROVE SHOULDER STABILITY

Neutral Rotation: Stand with your left side toward a cable pulley station. Grasp the handle in your right hand and begin with your right arm bent 90 degrees across your belly so that your forearm is pointing toward the cable pulley station.

Rotate your shoulder to pull the handle across your body. Return to the starting position. Complete 10 repetitions, then turn and repeat the exercise with your left arm.

Overhead Rotation: Stand with your right upper arm extended away from your body at shoulder level, your elbow bent 90 degrees and your shoulder rotated internally so your forearm is pointing toward the floor. Hold a small dumbbell in your right hand.

Rotate your shoulder externally 180 degrees, stopping when your right forearm is pointing toward the ceiling. Return to the starting position. Complete 10 repetitions, then repeat the exercise with your left arm.

Chapter 2

The Morning-After Problem

Among the universal experiences in the running community is something called *delayed-onset muscle soreness (DOMS)*, a somewhat elaborate way of saying "muscle stiffness." This is the characteristic pain that reduces you to a shuffle the day after your first run or a harder run than usual.

Even the most experienced runners endure DOMS after intense running—or any other activity, for that matter—that their bodies are not used to. This is a part of running that we'd all love to avoid, but it lies in wait for us after hard training. It is the morning-after problem.

Introducing DOMS: The Most Feared Acronym in Running

You may recall your first foray into the world of running, when you went from zero to, perhaps, four miles on your first jog and felt pretty good about it. No sooner had you showered than you were looking forward to the next run. After a good night's rest, you woke up the next morning expecting to jump out of bed ready to tackle the day. Instead, your reward for completing those four miles was an inability to move your legs! Your muscles, especially your quads and calves, were almost paralyzed by pain and tenderness. You got out of bed in four separate movements, gently levering yourself up and holding on to the wall as you made your way to the bathroom.

For the next two days, the pain got progressively worse, which you could only imagine must mean the worst: You must be injured. After all, you reasoned, a few aches and pains were to be expected, but a progressive increase in pain over 72 hours certainly was not in the plan.

Then, almost as stealthily as it emerged, the pain began to subside. You no longer had to modify your movements, and you were able to walk normally. Stairs still hurt, but after another day or so, that was fine too, and you were ready for your next run. So you laced up your shoes, not entirely without trepidation (once bitten, twice shy), and headed out for another run, making sure to keep this one "gentle."

The next morning, you woke up anticipating your four-phase bed dismount—but there was no pain. Perhaps some discomfort, but it was not limiting. By later that morning, it was almost gone, not to return until you got carried away again and asked your muscles to do more than they were up for.

This story, and any of its many possible variations, introduces a number of key characteristics that help us to understand what causes DOMS. But it's by no means the only scenario in which DOMS develops.

Consider whether you can relate to any of the following:

→ You are an experienced runner who, after a layoff from running (due to work, injury, weather, or motivation), decides to resume and head out for what used to be your typical run. You wake up the next morning with a pain you thought was no longer possible, given your running history.

→ After months of training, you complete your first marathon feeling tired but strong, then you wake up the next day completely incapacitated by pain. Did you just not train enough?

→ Friends take you on a new route through the trails, with numerous sections of steep up- and downhills and even some stairs. Though it's half the length of your usual road run, the next day your legs feel as though they've exploded. Are you injured? Or were you just weak?

→ You're a regular runner, but you've decided to introduce a bit of variety in your plan, so you attend a yoga class with a friend. The next day, the other participants are bouncing around, while you nurse your aching limbs back to health for a week.

Such stories are common, and they share a common theme—DOMS. The stimulus is slightly different, and the context of each is of course different, but we're sure that every reader of this book will have recognized at least one of these scenarios from personal—and possibly painful—experience.

Our objective is to explain what is happening physiologically in these scenarios, so that you can fully understand DOMS and the means to prevent it.

THE DOMS MYTHS: WHAT IT IS NOT

The first study describing a potential cause of muscle soreness after exercise was published in 1902. It suggested that the pain was caused by microscopic tears in the muscle fibers. According to Priscilla Clarkson, one of the world's leading authorities on DOMS, research lost impetus some time after that, and in the 10-year period from 1970 to 1980, only five studies on DOMS were published. Research on the phenomenon has grown exponentially since then, with more than 100 studies published in the past 10 years. Despite new studies and the fact that someone was on to the true cause more than 100 years ago (as we'll see shortly), numerous myths about the possible cause of DOMS have infiltrated the popular media. Perhaps a good starting point is to explain what we know does *not* cause DOMS.

The Scientific Process: Shooting the Wrong Messenger

To understand how the DOMS myth evolved, you must recognize that any scientist is only as good as his eyes. In other words, it is possible to understand and explain only what can be observed. When direct observation is not possible, the next best thing is to infer cause and effect by linking two related observations (provided, of course, that the link is not completely arbitrary).

This logic, which is universally applied, often with incorrect results, says that if we know that A causes B, and that A also causes C, then B *might* be responsible for C. Applying this thinking to DOMS, scientists and runners very quickly recognized that a hard running session (A) caused muscle pain the next morning (B), especially if the runner was not accustomed to it. The next step was to identify variable C, and the first likely candidate that emerged was a molecule called lactate.

Produced as a result of metabolic processes that generate energy for your muscles, lactate has received perhaps the worst reputation of any molecule in all of exercise physiology. It has not only been "in the dock" for muscle damage, but has also been falsely accused of causing fatigue and muscle pain during running. Why has lactate been so falsely fingered? Because lactate was one of the first metabolic "by-products" of exercise to be identified, as far back as the 1930s. It was easy to measure, and its levels changed in response to a variety of exercise situations. It wasn't immediately named lactate, but its bad reputation grew when scientists discovered that:

→ Lactate was formed when muscle was denied oxygen. Insufficient oxygen was always deemed to be the crucial limitation to exercise performance; the increased production of lactate was perceived as very convincing evidence of its role in the fatigue process.

→ Lactate was produced in greater quantities during faster-paced running.

Since faster-paced running is also more likely to cause muscle fatigue and muscle damage, lactate's candidacy as the intermediary (C) in the muscle damage explanation was strengthened. Pretty soon, lactate was equated with "exercise poison," and the pain felt by runners the day after running was lumped together with the many other detrimental effects lactate produced.

We'll discuss lactate in much greater detail in Chapter 8, which covers metabolism and fatigue, but for our present objective, suffice it to say that the basic theory for DOMS was that an uncharacteristic running session (A) caused DOMS (B) as a result of lactate formation (C). This myth gained even greater traction when coaches and athletes learned that if the athlete jogged lightly at the end of a hard session, he or she could reduce the severity of the muscle pain somewhat. The theory was that the light jogging helped "flush" out the lactate, thereby attenuating the pain it would otherwise cause. Simple enough, but as we shall see, quite incorrect on all counts.

When it comes to lactate and DOMS, scientific breakthroughs resulted from an improvement in the ability to "see" the muscle. The invention of the muscle biopsy technique, in which a small piece of muscle is taken from an athlete and then examined under a powerful microscope, revealed a whole new angle to DOMS.

In 1981, a Swedish scientist named Jan Friden published research findings. He asked volunteers to walk repeatedly down a flight of stairs and took a biopsy of their muscle afterward. His observations provided some of the first evidence of the real cause of DOMS, and we'll tackle them shortly.

However, this scientific study was slow to make an impact on the general public, and the lactate theory persisted as the cause of postexercise muscle soreness in popular media, running magazines, and coaching circles. In true detective style, then, consider the following questions about DOMS, based on your own experience of running, because the answers will steer us away from the lactate red herring, toward the real answer.

Q *What type of running causes the most severe DOMS?*

A Any experienced runner will tell you that DOMS is much more severe after very long distance runs at a slow pace or after very fast-paced running, such as speed workouts or hill training. The lactate theory does fit with the experience of DOMS after faster running, because more lactate is produced at faster speeds. But what of long, slow running? Ultramarathon runners know that no amount of training will prevent DOMS from occurring after events, virtually regardless of how slowly they run. The lactate theory of DOMS does not fit with this experience, because lactate forms in significant amounts only when we run faster, and most marathon or ultramarathon runners finish having produced very little lactate, yet they can still barely get out of bed after an event.

You may also know from experience that DOMS is particularly severe if you run downhill or do a series of jumping exercises. In the laboratory, there is a protocol for causing DOMS, in which volunteers jump off a 1-meter-high box 100 times. Most dismiss this task as very easy, laughing their way through it, until the next day, when they can barely walk. Again, very little lactate is formed during these jumps, and lactate production is also lower during downhill running than during normal, level-road running. Yet both cause much more severe muscle pain than running either uphill or on a level surface.

Finally, this discussion revolves around the kind of running that will lead to DOMS, which suggests a significant question—why does cycling not cause the same degree of muscle damage and DOMS as running? The lactate levels produced during very hard cycling are at least comparable to those of running, but the DOMS is nowhere near as severe, suggesting that something in the act of running, and not a common chemical, is to blame.

Q *When does DOMS occur?*

A The first scenario we depicted at the beginning of this chapter is typical of DOMS—no problem during the run, but 12 to 24 hours later, the pain starts and then builds progressively during the day. Research has shown that the most severe pain tends to occur between 24 and 72 hours after exercise. Given that lactate levels are back to normal within 30 minutes of exercise, it's difficult to see how lactate could directly cause stiffness and pain. It could, of course, set in motion a sequence of events leading to the pain, but the fact that the pain lasts for up to three days, by which time lactate is long removed and forgotten, suggests there is a much more complex process in play.

Q *What other kinds of activities cause DOMS?*

A Runners often believe themselves to be among the fittest people around, often rightly so. Yet running fitness doesn't always translate well into other activities—a reality that is often made painfully apparent the day after exercise in an unfamiliar activity, when DOMS emerges as the surest sign that fitness is sport-specific and "contextual." A runner who ventures onto a tennis court, into the weight room, even into a yoga studio for the first time is likely to be humbled for a couple of days afterward with aching and stiff muscles. These activities typically produce less lactate than a running session, yet they can cause very severe DOMS. Even stretching causes DOMS, if it is overdone, in what is one of the most telling clues to the real cause. Of course, stretching produces almost no lactate, so an alternative explanation must be sought.

Exceptions to the Rules: Time to Change the Theory

In science, when exceptions to the theory or results that cannot be explained by the prevailing theory are discovered, the prevailing theory might be in need of revision. Until the turn of the 16th century, for example, it was thought that only white swans existed. However, the discovery of a black swan in Australia proved the consensus about swan color incorrect, and the paradigm needed change. The existence of even a single black swan rendered all previous theories and ideas about its impossibility invalid. As it turned out, black swans were numerous; you just had to look in the right place for them. This concept is the framework for Nassim Nicholas Talieb's book *The Black Swan*, but it's also relevant to our DOMS discussion. The three just-discussed questions demonstrate that lactate, often thought in public circles to be the answer to muscle stiffness, fails to explain DOMS in any instance.

These three situations are the black swans of DOMS theory, and so it is time to adjust the theory of the likely cause of DOMS, aided by powerful electron microscopes and a dose of basic physiology, courtesy of Hans Selye.

MUSCLE SORENESS AND OVERLOAD: LESSONS FROM HANS SELYE

In the introduction to this book, we presented the General Adaptation Principle of scientist Hans Selye and explained how the management of training stress is the single most important factor determining your running success. You have to control the training load so that you are stressed enough to adapt but not so stressed that your physiological capacity to adapt is exhausted, which we know will lead to injury or overtraining.

This model can easily be applied to muscle soreness. Muscle is a living, dynamic, and continuously changing tissue that adapts to training by increasing (or decreasing) the size of its fibers, as well as their number and internal functions.

So what do Hans Selye and his Adaptation Principle tell us about DOMS? On first consideration, it would seem that the pain associated with DOMS is anything but adaptation. It feels more like the first stage of injury, especially because the pain gets worse and worse over the course of the first 48 hours after training. However, recall from the Selye model that the body's first response to an applied stress is the "alarm reaction." DOMS is nothing more than the alarm reaction to a bout of exercise that is more stressful than the muscles are familiar with.

Taking a more long-term view, DOMS is actually part of a process that will lead you into a stage of adaptation, in which running is easier, the muscles are stronger, and DOMS is (thankfully) a distant memory. We therefore need to consider how DOMS ultimately results in an overall improvement in muscle strength and in the ability to withstand further bouts of exercise.

THE PHYSIOLOGY OF DOMS: A COMPLEX PROCESS WITH A SIMPLE OUTCOME

Running is perceived as a stressor for many reasons. To allow you to run around the block, let alone complete an easy six-mile jog, your body performs an incredible range of physiological feats. The faster or farther you run, of course, the greater the stress response necessary to allow you to finish. And that stress response often endures after the run, as is the case with DOMS. There are thus two distinct phases in the DOMS process—the actual stress phase and the subsequent response that "corrects" the changes caused by exercise, which happens, at the same time, to be responsible for your pain.

Phase 1: Eccentric Muscle Contraction and Structural Damage to Muscle

We've already made the observation that cycling produces very little DOMS, regardless of how hard you ride, whereas even an easy run can cause major soreness the morning after. The difference between cycling and running, of course, is impact. Specifically, the eccentric muscle contractions of running point to the mechanism behind DOMS. Eccentric muscle contractions are those in which the muscle has to decelerate the limb by contracting against an external load. Put more technically, the load torque exceeds the muscle torque, and the result is that work is done *on* the muscle, which lengthens as it contracts (one of the more bizarre oxymorons in exercise physiology). This happens every time your foot hits the ground—the muscles contract in order to decelerate the leg, working against gravity to stabilize the joints and keep them from buckling.

During this process, the muscle becomes damaged, because your muscle fibers are literally pulled apart under load every single time you strike the ground—a 30-minute run entails about 2,600 "pulls" on each leg. Imagine a piece of elastic that is constantly being stretched under a heavy load. After 2,600 stretches, that elastic is very likely to be close to breaking. You can appreciate how your muscle is being exposed to enormous forces every time you land. It's obvious that your muscles are doing an incredible job to allow you to run at all.

You can also appreciate that the weaker the piece of elastic, the sooner it will break, so weaker muscle fibers will begin to be structurally damaged by the constant loading. This is precisely what happens when you run—the tiny myofibrils, made up of myosin and actin are actually pulled apart, causing damage inside the muscle cell at a microscopic level.

When damaged muscle is viewed under a microscope with sufficient resolution, the results are plain to see.

Viewing the undamaged muscle alongside the damaged sample makes one think of a nicely assembled brick wall, where the bricks comprise neatly arranged *sarcomeres*, the structural units of striated muscle fibrils.

The damaged muscle, however, looks as if it were exposed to an earthquake that left the ordered structure looking somewhat shaken, if still standing (barely). To get technical, the disordered structure is characterized by what scientists call Z-line streaming. The Z-lines, which normally anchor the ends of the sarcomeres, are now "streaming," no longer holding the symmetrical, bricklike structures in place. Streaming is a sign that the entire scaffolding that holds the muscle together has been damaged by the eccentric contractions. That is the root problem, and the next step, performed by your body, is to repair and then regenerate.

Phase 2: Damage Repair

So far, we've established that the "morning-after" pain you feel is the result of structural damage to the muscle. That's hardly reassuring! After all, who wants to know that the act of running is damaging muscles, ripping the myofibrils apart with every stride? That would seem a reason to avoid running, if ever there was one.

Well, all is not lost. The good news is that the body responds to this structural damage with a process that ultimately produces a stronger, more durable muscle. Just as a structural engineer will arrive after an earthquake and clear the damage, reinforce a building's foundations, and then create a more solid, damage-resistant structure, the body responds by "cleaning up the damage" and rebuilding, producing muscle fibers that are far more capable of withstanding the stress the next time.

This process is, unfortunately, also responsible for your pain and discomfort in the next few days, but it's a small price to pay for more resilient muscle in the future. The process varies quite widely, depending on the intensity of the exercise, the type of exercise that caused the damage, and the individual, but it generally plays out as follows.

THE INFLAMMATORY RESPONSE AND MUSCLE DAMAGE

The initial mechanical trauma and damage to the muscle structure initiate what is known as the inflammatory response. Fluid and cells move to the damaged muscle and infiltrate the tissue. The first of these cells are thought to be *neutrophils* and *macrophages*, which are circulating in your blood as you read this. These cells go about destroying the dead tissue, clearing away damaged cells. They do this by literally "digesting" those damaged cells (a process called phagocytosis), and by releasing enzymes and oxygen molecules that degrade that tissue.

This degradation can be quite indiscriminate—it doesn't really single out only damaged cells. It can therefore cause further muscle damage, which may seem somewhat counterintuitive, but recall that the first objective of reconstruction is to clear away the debris and rubble to create a "clean space" for rebuilding. Neutrophils and macrophages are the bulldozers and dump trucks of your body, clearing away the rubble to make it easier to rebuild later on.

The neutrophils perform another important function: They signal other inflammatory cells to move to the area. One such cell is a *monocyte*, which enters the muscle and continues the process of degrading and digesting the damaged muscle tissue. Monocytes release chemicals known as *cytokines*, which can either increase or reduce the inflammatory process. This is because two types of cytokines exist: pro-inflammatory and anti-inflammatory cytokines. The balance between these two chemicals is important because it is thought to create a compromise between the requirement to heal the muscle through inflammation and the need to prevent excessive inflammation, which would damage the muscle even more. To extend our building analogy, too many bulldozers would destroy everything; too few and you'd be rebuilding on a damaged foundation. So balance is the key.

All these chemicals at the site of muscle damage cause the muscle membrane to become leaky. This has two effects. The first is to allow certain enzymes to escape from inside the muscle. One of these, *creatine kinase*, is an indicator chemical and is often measured in the blood as a signal that muscle damage has occurred. The second effect is that fluid can move into the muscle. This causes swelling. If you ever have a bad case of DOMS, you might measure the circumference of the painful muscle and find that it is much larger than normal. The swelling causes pressure to build inside the tissue, and this is thought to be the primary source of your pain, especially when you move suddenly, asking that swollen muscle to contract—it pushes against nerve endings, causing more pain than normal.

To make matters even worse, other chemicals, called prostaglandins, histamines, and bradykinins (a mouthful, admittedly), are released when tissue is damaged, and they are thought to make the nerve endings more sensitive to stimulation. Your nerve endings, therefore, are highly sensitive. They might have been slightly damaged themselves by the exercise and subsequent inflammation and are now being compressed by a swollen muscle. It's little wonder that you struggle to walk down the stairs the morning after a marathon. This pain has a protective function, however, since it discourages you from doing any further damage to the muscles.

All the while, the muscle has begun its own regenerative process. Those dead cells, which are so ably being cleared out by the neutrophils, macrophages, and monocytes, are gradually being replaced by new muscle cells. Again, it's important to remove all the cellular debris so that the new cells can be laid down on a clean foundation, and this is what happens. Cells known as *satellite cells* move to the damaged area—Think of them as the bricklayers in this reconstruction process. They finish the job by actually laying down new muscle fibers; fibers can either fuse to existing muscle cells or be converted into entirely new cells, which results in a new population of potentially stronger, more capable muscle fibers.

This entire process—which is clearly complex—first removes damaged tissue, then repairs the area, and finally regenerates the muscle fiber population. The pain is an unfortunate side effect of the process, but it's clear now why your pain arrives the morning after—all these processes take a few hours to start working, and the swelling and inflammation peak 24 to 48 hours after damage.

PROTECTED IN THE LONG RUN

The good news is that this pain is not in vain. The old saying "No pain, no gain" is appropriate here, because the eventual outcome of this entire process is that your muscles become stronger, and less likely to be damaged in the future. Scientific studies have shown that for up to six months, a second bout of potentially damaging exercise will cause far less DOMS than the first. This is known as the *repeat bout effect.*

The mechanism is not well understood, however. One theory is that there are neural factors which allow for more efficient recruitment patterns as a result of training. According to this theory, your body learns how to activate muscle fibers more effectively so that you spread the load more evenly the second time around, causing less damage per muscle fiber. This theory is probably only a part of the answer, however. It's more likely that the simple "survival of the fittest" principle explains why you become immune to DOMS with a bit of training.

From this perspective, what happens is that the first run causes damage to the muscle fibers, with the weakest fibers being damaged first and most severely. Once the repair and regeneration process is complete, the weaker fibers have either been destroyed and replaced or rebuilt stronger than before, leaving behind a population of much more resistant muscle fibers. Think of that first training session as the team tryouts that sift out the weaker players. Once the repair process is complete, all that remain are the stronger fibers, and hence future exercise doesn't cause muscle damage or DOMS. If, however, you abruptly run much faster or farther than normal, then you're again overtaxing your relatively weaker fibers, and the body has to respond by clearing them out. There is therefore a constant cycle of damage and repair. The trick is to maintain the balance so that you don't ever cause damage beyond repair, which we'll discuss at the end of the chapter.

APPRECIATE THE MORNING AFTER

Now that we've explained the likely cause of your DOMS, we're in a far better position to answer the three questions we asked earlier in this chapter, which lactate was unable to explain:

Q *What type of running causes the most severe DOMS?*

A Sprinting causes DOMS because muscle is being asked to contract at incredibly high rates, under enormous forces that it may be unaccustomed to, even in experienced runners. The first speedwork sessions of a season always cause pain the day after, because the weaker muscle fibers are not able to handle the load they are placed under.

Similarly, slow distance running is far more likely to cause DOMS because of the sheer number of contractions, particularly eccentric contractions, and the fact that fatigued muscle is less able to cope with the repeated demands to resist the forces of gravity made by every single footstrike. Therefore, the stress is a function of the intensity of contraction (in sprinting) and the total volume (in long-

distance running) of contraction. Finally, downhill running causes much more severe DOMS because the eccentric contractions of the muscle are far more forceful when you run downhill—the jarring effect you perceive on a steep descent is to blame.

Q *When does DOMS occur?*

A We can now appreciate why DOMS is most severe between 24 and 48 hours after the actual run. This is the time required for all the regenerative processes to kick into gear. The swelling, sensitization of the nerve endings, and chemical breakdown of damaged tissue take a while to run their course. This confirms that it's not the actual act of running that causes the pain but rather the process by which the running-induced damage is repaired.

Q *What other kinds of activities cause DOMS?*

A We can also appreciate why you, the runner, will struggle with DOMS after trying your hand at a new activity. Your legs, accustomed to many hours of straight-ahead, running-related contraction, are suddenly asked to contract in a completely different manner. Playing tennis, for example, asks a whole new group of muscles to work, while the same muscles must now work quite differently. (Your quads and hamstrings suddenly have to stop you, change your direction, and so on.) The arms, meanwhile, that you may never give a second thought to are suddenly working both eccentrically and concentrically, and some pain the day after is the inevitable result. If you venture into the gym for the first time in months and do some resistance training, you'll experience the most extreme example of this phenomenon. And you now know that it's not so much lifting the weights as lowering them back down that is the source of your pain, because this is when the eccentric phase of the contraction occurs.

As for stretching and yoga, the simple act of stretching the muscle causes the same kind of process to occur: muscle damage, followed by a process of repair and regeneration. The mechanism is different, but the resulting process and final outcome are similar.

MANAGEMENT AND PREVENTION

All this knowledge and understanding is worth very little if we cannot prevent DOMS from happening more than necessary and manage it better when it does occur.

Preventing DOMS: Better Than a Cure

Prevention is always better than a cure, so any steps that can be taken to prevent DOMS are desirable. Recall that DOMS is the symptom of the process by which muscle damage is repaired; therefore, in this case, *prevention means preventing muscle damage, not the symptoms after the damage has occurred.* Once the muscle is damaged, it is in a sense too late to

intervene, and the focus should shift to managing the repair process, which we'll discuss shortly.

So, how do we prevent the damage from occurring to begin with? Unfortunately, complete prevention is not compatible with your desire to become a better runner. If you want to improve as a runner, then part of the deal is that your weaker muscles need to be strengthened. This objective is achieved only through the process of stress and adaptation, so some muscle damage is part of the bargain. You'll never sift out those weaker fibers if you don't accept this reality. Trying to avoid muscle damage is akin to trying to train without ever breathing harder or raising your heart rate above about 100 beats per minute. You can do it, but you'll never really improve.

However, there is no reason why your first run or training program needs to leave you partially paralyzed for three days. There are means to reduce the severity of the muscle damage and resultant DOMS. As we've seen, it's all about managing the stress—controlling that alarm reaction. We spoke earlier of the repeat bout effect, in which the body adapts to exercise so that a second running session doesn't cause nearly the same degree of DOMS as the first. The good news is that this repeat bout effect seems to exist even when the first run doesn't cause DOMS. In other words, you become resistant to muscle damage without ever actually damaging the muscle. You don't have to go out and run yourself into a DOMS-induced partial paralysis in order to benefit from the body's adaptations. It seems that even a mild bout of exercise, a very easy run, is able to produce the same overall adaptive responses that protect you from DOMS later on.

Therefore, the simplest (yet undoubtedly most difficult to achieve) solution is to do your first run at a level that is well below your normal expectation of your running ability. Don't go out and run six miles on your first training run; rather, do three miles, and mix slow jogging with brisk walking. You might feel as if you're wasting your time, but scientific studies have shown that even this easy training will protect against DOMS after future runs. You might, for your second run, increase the distance to about 75 percent of what you think your typical distance will be, and ease your way into the program step-by-step thereafter. Most runners never do this and begin at a gallop, but simply setting aside perhaps one week to ease your way into training will almost completely prevent the DOMS problem later on.

You can also control the impact factor by running a few sessions on softer surfaces, such as grass and gravel. Also, avoiding excessive downhill running in the first week or two of a new running season will help prevent muscle damage.

Finally, we've mentioned that the weaker muscle fibers are the most easily damaged under the load of running, so a key strategy is to strengthen the muscle. Many runners have little time for strength work in the gym, but if performance is your buzzword and avoiding DOMS is important, then time in the gym or doing body-weight training at home is crucial. Of course, you are just as much at risk of muscle damage the first time you go to the gym, so the same principle applies—start at a very easy level, giving your muscles a good week to adapt. Lift light weights, do few repetitions, and avoid reaching muscle fatigue or strain. In good time, you'll have adapted enough to ramp up the training and start cashing in without DOMS-inducing damage. This approach is particularly important for runners who focus heavily on speedwork and can't afford to sit out three days after every tough session because their muscles are too sore to run.

There may be good reason to want to prevent severe DOMS from happening repeatedly (apart from the obvious pain the next morning, that is). There was, until relatively recently, some thought that the regeneration and repair of muscle fibers after damage was exhaustible. In other words, you had a limited capacity to repair damaged muscle, and there would come a time when your satellite cell population would diminish, meaning your "muscle-making account" could be depleted if you suffered DOMS once too often.

World-famous heart surgeon Dr. Christian Barnard once said that the heart has a finite number of contractions in its life span; if this theory applied, running would be dangerous, because you'd use up your allocation far sooner if you ran regularly. Thankfully, Dr. Barnard was wrong, and there is now a growing body of thought that the theory of limited muscle repair is also incorrect. However, the jury is still out, with the experts debating the issue as you read this. So the safe approach, which is quite achievable, is to control training to prevent excessive DOMS whenever possible.

If you can just get past the initial stress of running, you will reduce the severity of the alarm reaction but still benefit from the adaptations in the muscle that can make you stronger in the future.

Managing DOMS:
Let the Process Happen

Prevention is not always possible, or even desirable, in the case of muscle damage, since it's the catalyst for strengthening the muscles. Therefore some degree of DOMS is inevitable, regardless of your strategy to prevent it. Once the inevitable happens, the key is to recognize that the process taking place is beneficial in the long term, so you could do a lot worse than stand aside and let that natural process happen. There is often a fine line between interfering with what is a crucially important process of regeneration and managing it so that it works optimally, while relieving yourself of some of the discomfort at the same time.

The worst thing you can do is to try to interfere with the process by using medical products. Many runners don't react drastically to DOMS and choose instead to recog-

nize the funny side of the situation, waiting out the time in self-inflicted discomfort. However, the liberal use of pain medication anti-inflammatories and other treatments to alleviate the pain is still relatively common. Recall that the pain is a symptom caused by inflammation, swelling, and the presence of chemicals that make the nerves more sensitive. If you take anti-inflammatories to prevent the swelling and pain, then you are in effect preventing your body's natural bulldozers from clearing out a damaged area so that new, stronger muscle can be laid down.

We mentioned earlier that excessive inflammation can cause even more damage, and that is why some people do advocate the use of anti-inflammatories for injuries, leading to a lively debate in academic and medical circles about when anti-inflammatories should or should not be used.

The general consensus regarding anti-inflammatories and injuries—and DOMS is included in this category—is that the initial inflammation is very important for repair and recovery, and only much later, after many days, should the inflammation be controlled so as to prevent excessive damage. In the case of DOMS, when the pain will last only a few days, prolonged inflammation is unlikely, so the use of anti-inflammatories is likely to hinder rather than help the process and should be avoided.

As for the range of products that are sold to prevent muscle soreness, they have by now (hopefully) been debunked. These include gels and creams that supposedly reduce the production of lactate, which, as we've seen, has nothing to do with DOMS anyway. There are other creams, many herbal-based, that supposedly act in an anti-inflammatory manner. They should probably be avoided, for the reasons explained earlier. The best thing to do, apart from avoiding excessive training when you begin your program, is to ride out the pain and learn from your experience, so that you limit the degree of damage in the future.

One method that has been found to help a little, at least in terms of reducing the severity of the DOMS, is to finish hard running sessions with a light jog. You'll recall that coaches and athletes made this observation and incorrectly attributed it to the assumption that the slow jogging would help clear the lactate faster. That's not the reason, and science doesn't really know why this practice of easy jogging might work, but it seems, based on the experience of runners, to do so. It's not always practical, of course; if you've just done a 20-mile training run at an already easy pace, the addition of another mile of slow jogging is probably going to worsen, rather than improve, your symptoms. But after track workouts and hard hill sessions, it is worth trying—and it does have other benefits, so there's little to lose.

One final note on letting the process happen is never to do any hard training when you have DOMS. Part of the process is allowing your body to manage this sequence of inflammation and repair without inducing any further stress. So if you have DOMS, a couple of days of rest is best. If you really feel that you must get a run in to stay sane, then it must be a dawdle!

In any case, there is much scientific evidence to show that when damaged enough to produce DOMS, your muscles lose some of their strength. Therefore, any hard running you try to do will not be very high quality. So take it easy and use the one to two days of rest to catch up on something else in your life while your muscles and body do their thing. Percy Cerutty, the famous Australian running coach who counted John Landy and Herb Elliott among his athletes, once said, "Pain is the purifier. Love pain. Embrace pain."

It would be asking the impossible to tell you that you should embrace the pain of DOMS. But hopefully you now recognize that muscle damage happens because unprepared muscle fibers are asked to do work they're not ready for. The process by which the damage is repaired is the cause of your pain, but it's also the first step toward becoming a better runner. So while you may never *embrace* the pain of the morning after, you will perhaps recognize that it is not all bad, and that once the curtain of pain is lifted, you're better off for it.

It is important, however, to manage your training to avoid DOMS as much as you reasonably can. The simple act of managing that initial stress so that it doesn't cause too great an alarm reaction goes a long way toward getting the best of both worlds: minimal pain, with the same gain—adaptation.

Chapter 3

Big Impact

NASA's finest structural engineers would be hard-pressed to design a material like your bone. The specifications of bone, given its functions in your body, read like those for a high-tech material the likes of which you expect to see in a fictional Hollywood movie. Bone is responsible for supporting enormous loads over a prolonged period and must therefore be both strong and resilient; it cannot be too stiff, since the risk of fracture would increase, nor too flexible, since structural stability would be compromised. It is able to withstand up to 100,000 impact forces of up to six times your body weight per week. Carried around for 24 hours a day, it must be extremely light so that transportation is not a physical impossibility. Oh, and it has to be alive, so that it is able to adapt to the demands being placed on it by becoming stronger and quite literally changing its structure on a constant basis. To cap it all off, it must have a life span of 70 or more years!

Those "specifications" describe what bone is capable of—it is the living high-tech material that makes up our skeletons and that we take for granted, until such time as it "fails" and the material doesn't withstand the excessive loads we place on it.

And fail it does. Unfortunately, many running injuries are the result of the failure of bone to adapt to the stresses of running. The incidence of stress fractures, one of the more common running injuries, in which the bone develops tiny fractures along its length, is reported to be as high as 20 percent. In the next chapter, we'll discover a model that explains these injuries, and we'll see how the principle of adaptation to stress can help you avoid the stress that would cause fractures in your bones.

A more generalized problem, however, is a condition known as osteoporosis, which is characterized by weakened bones that result from very low bone mineral density (BMD) and which affects mostly women (for reasons we'll get into later). There are different classifications of the condition. At its mildest, it is called osteopenia. Osteoporosis is a step more severe than this. Finally, severe osteoporosis is diagnosed when there is evidence of fractures.

People with osteoporosis have very fragile skeletons, and they are likely to suffer fractures extremely easily. Simple acts that normal bones are more than capable of handling many times over are now enough to precipitate traumatic fractures.

Osteoporosis did not even register on doctors' view screens 25 years ago, but today is recognized as an epidemic as a result of the fractures it causes, which cost the medical industry billions of dollars per year. The sudden "explosion" in the condition is not entirely real—much of it is perceived, driven by increased awareness, better testing methods and equipment to measure bone mineral density, and the fact that more people are being educated about bone health. You probably know people who have this condition, who have perhaps experienced fractures as a result.

The good news is that as a runner, you have an upper hand in the fight against osteoporosis, because the impact of running can be a positive stress that helps your bones adapt and become stronger. If you are not a runner (yet), you can also take heart because taking up running will help you increase BMD and strengthen your bones, regardless of when you start. And finally, if you already have osteopenia or osteoporosis, there's good news for you as well. There is some evidence, which we'll devote some time to in this chapter, that BMD increases when those with already weakened bones start a well-designed exercise program that includes some strength training and walking and jogging. Of course, you have to be careful not to overdo it, perhaps more than most, but with the right approach, there's no doubt that exercise training helps anyone, regardless of their age, gender, and current bone health.

Understanding Bone: A Living Material

At a very basic level, bone consists of three components: water, an organic component, and an inorganic component. The organic component of bone is composed of ground substance and collagen, which we introduced when discussing muscle and tendon; and cells, which control the function of the bone. Collagen, a protein, is the main structural component of bone. A long protein fibril, collagen is grouped with other collagen fibrils to form a large fiber, much as muscle is constructed of small fibrils coming together to form a fiber. The function-regulating cells are *osteoblasts*, *osteocytes*, and *osteoclasts*, which we'll cover when we address the adaptations of bone to the mechanical stresses of running.

Bone stores 98 percent of your body's calcium. The inorganic component of bone is effectively your body's storage repository for calcium and phosphate. These two minerals combine to form a crystal known as hydroxyapatite, which is the main component of the inorganic component of bone. Crystals of hydroxyapatite are packed into bone around and between the collagen fibers, and they provide the mineral constituents that give bone a substantial part of its strength, which is why you've always heard that getting calcium in your diet through dairy helps build strong bones.

Teamwork—How Cells Shift the Balance of Your Bone

Rather than focus primarily on the anatomy of bone, we'll consider how bone responds to stressors such as running and the impact associated with your feet striking the ground, which transmits up to six times your body weight through your bones per landing. But in order to understand this response, we have to understand a few basics about how bone cells function, constantly changing the balance between bone breakdown and bone formation, which is happening in your bones even as you read this.

First are the osteoblasts. These tiny cells are responsible for producing what is called bone matrix—the collagen and ground substance. Osteoblasts are living cells, controlled by hormones and other chemicals, which position themselves on the bone wherever bone formation is required. Their job is to produce the organic component of bone, which is followed by the calcification process.

Once this process is completed, the osteoblasts become osteocytes, or mature bone cells, which are embedded inside the bone, or calcified. Calcification of bone is the physiological equivalent of a cement truck being buried inside its own construction site as the cement hardens around it. The osteocytes are all connected to one another by long processes, forming something of a web of bone cells that helps them to communicate with one another and initiate the bone's collective response to stressors such as mechanical loading.

The third type of cell is an osteoclast, which is responsible for the removal of bone, a process called resorption. Osteoclasts are the body's equivalent of wrecking balls, though their function is not quite as indiscriminate as this analogy would suggest. They work by releasing enzymes onto the bone, which dissolve the calcium component of bone. Other enzymes join in to remove the collagen part of bone.

It should not surprise you to learn that the activities of the osteoblasts (the bone-forming units) and the osteoclasts (the bone resorption units) are very closely linked. Your body switches on bone resorption only after bone formation has finished, so that the two follow one another very closely. They are also linked in magnitude—if one increases, the other follows suit, which is sensible given the importance of maintaining the balance of bone mass.

The processes in which bone structure is constantly altered by the balance of activity between the osteoblasts and the osteoclasts are called *modeling* and *remodeling*. Modeling happens when bone cell activity is controlled to change the bone's strength and structure and allow growth by sending osteoblasts and osteoclasts to specific locations on the bone. Think of a potter working clay with her hands and changing the shape—that's modeling.

Bone remodeling, on the other hand, is of more interest to you, the runner. This is the step-by-step activation of osteoclasts and then osteoblasts to prevent and repair fatigue damage to the bone. For example, when an area of bone has been overloaded or is damaged at a microscopic level, the remodeling process kicks into gear to repair the damage. If this strikes you as similar in concept to the process by which muscle damage is repaired, you're right—in principle, anyway. The damage is healed first by removal of bone by osteoclasts and then by replacement of equal amounts of bone by the osteoblasts.

However, with aging, osteoporosis, and excessive training, the balance between bone resorption and bone formation may be disrupted. The result is that resorption becomes dominant. When this happens, the bone is not fully replaced, bone mass is lost, and the strength and integrity of the skeleton are reduced. This is obviously not a good situation, so it's important to understand how bone responds to the stress of training to ensure that we remain in bone balance.

Under Stress—The Impact of Impact on Bone

Mechanotransduction and Wolff's Law are fancy terms that explain how bone is able to sense and then respond to the stress of impact. Every physical activity, and running in particular (since it produces repeated high-impact forces), causes force to be applied to the skeleton.

The cells react to this force application by a process of mechanotransduction, which changes the balance between formation and resorption. It works because the osteocytes (bone cells) are all connected to one another in a three-dimensional network that is able to sense exactly where and when bone is being loaded. Thanks to a complex mechanism that allows impact forces to be converted into chemical signals. The end result is that when bone is deformed by impact, osteoclasts and osteoblasts are sent to the appropriate areas to remove and then add bone to help strengthen it.

The whole bone, meanwhile, adapts to the impact by becoming stronger, according to something called Wolff's Law, reminiscent of an architect's credo that "form follows function." This law states that bone will optimize structure in order to withstand the loading on it. In other words, bone will adapt to loading stress by changing it's form, mass, and material properties as required.

The response of bone to stress is quite well understood. Stress is the force applied to the bone. As we've said, it can be as much as six times more than body weight per landing during running. Now think of slow-motion images you may have seen of a tennis ball or golf ball coming in contact with a tennis racket or golf club—the ball deforms substantially. That deformation is called strain. Bone is also deformed under stress.

Eventually, you reach failure, which is when the overstressed bone can no longer handle the stress being applied to it, and fractures result.

The explanation of the mechanical properties of bone is important for us to understand, because it helps us appreciate what the stress is that we are referring to when we talk about the adaptation of bone to loading. In a 10-mile run, you're going to stress each bone approximately 7,000 times. It's therefore vital that you don't load your bones beyond the yield region, as doing so will cause failure and injury. Therefore, in training, you have to manage stress, quite literally, by keeping the volume and impact down. Too much running early on, or too much faster-paced running at any time, will increase the overall stress on your bones, moving you nearer to the yield region and ultimately to a point of failure. This effect is exacerbated if the balance between bone removal and bone formation in the bone remodeling process is disrupted.

Understanding Exercise and Training for Bone Strength

Armed with the knowledge that your bone is alive and able to adapt to the stress of running, provided that you keep it within reasonable limits, your next questions are likely to be "What are those limits?" and "How do I manage my training to avoid bone stress injury?"

Unfortunately, the answers to these questions are not as simple as you might think. That's because the strength and resilience of your bones are dependent on a number of factors, including geometry (their shape), architecture (how the bone is put together at a cellular level), the size of the bone, and the factor that gets the most attention, the bone mineral content (BMC). The BMC provides a measure of the mass of the bone and accounts for perhaps 80 percent of its strength. It is also the easiest to measure using a technique called dual-energy X-ray absorptiometry (DEXA), and that is why it has attracted such focus as a key component of bone strength.

So as we turn our attention to how exercise affects bone health and strength, we'll focus on BMC, but bear in mind that exercise does alter all of the other variables as well.

The first and most important point to make about bone health and training is that regular running helps. It does so by preventing the decline in bone mass that is part of the aging process, as we'll discuss in more detail. The graph here is an illustrative representation of bone calcium content over the course of 70 years for both men and women. It shows clearly that peak bone mineral content is achieved between the ages of 20 and 30, after which follows a progressive decrease.

YOUNGER RUNNERS—
BEFORE THE PEAK

Regular running (and other physical activity) helps by increasing the peak in bone mineral content and also seems to slow the rate of decline after you hit your peak. For example, one study from the University of Saskatchewan tracked adolescents over a period of six years and found that peak bone mass was 9 percent (boys) and 17 percent (girls) higher in teens who were regularly active than for their inactive peers. Other studies have found similar relationships—as the hours of physical activity increase, bone strength, mass, and mineral content do, as well.

The bottom line is that the late teens and early 20s are the best "bone years" of your life, the time to get your bone mass as high as you can go before a long, (hopefully very) slow decline begins.

OLDER RUNNERS AND WOMEN WHO HAVE NOT YET REACHED MENOPAUSE

If you're already past the peak, there is still cause for optimism. Numerous studies have found that athletes have substantially more bone mineral than nonathletes and inactive control groups. This observation is not by itself proof of a causal connection, because it doesn't tell us anything about the bone mass of athletes before they became athletes. There's a chance that they started with denser bones in the first place and also that things like diet and other lifestyle habits (such as not smoking) that tend to accompany exercise explain much of the difference. To try to overcome some of these potential confounding factors, in a clever study method, scientists looked at the arms of tennis players. They found that the dominant playing arm has a mineral content that's roughly 5 percent greater than that of the weaker, nonplaying arm, suggesting that athletic use of a limb has a significant effect on the bones it stresses. The bottom line, though, is that if you're a regular runner, then there's a good chance that your bone density is a full 10 percent higher than that of inactive people. That's good news, regardless of the reasons.

Regular exercise defends or even increases BMC beyond the age of 30, whereas inactive people typically experience a decrease over

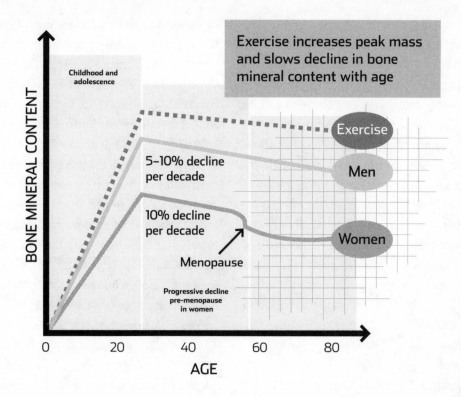

Exercise increases peak mass and slows decline in bone mineral content with age

BONE MINERAL CONTENT

Childhood and adolescence

Exercise

5–10% decline per decade

Men

10% decline per decade

Women

Menopause

Progressive decline pre-menopause in women

AGE

0   20   40   60   80

time. After around age 30, inactivity tends to be associated with a decline in BMD; the BMC difference between regular activity and inactivity grows to about 2 to 3 percent, mostly because you lose out when you're inactive. Taken collectively, it seems that you can expect roughly a 1 percent reversal of the normal, age-related loss in BMC per year if you exercise regularly. Running is a particularly good form of exercise because of the impact, which stimulates the adaptation process.

How long does the exercise program need to be maintained before it makes a measurable difference? That's not entirely clear; some studies find that increases in bone density reach a peak after 18 months, others that it happens within 6 to 9 months. The expert recommendation is that a program of exercise for bone health should last at least 9 months, preferably longer, and ideally for life. So if you're inspired to take up running, for your bones and other reasons, then you should commit for the long run, both literally and figuratively.

THE OLDER POPULATION AND POSTMENOPAUSAL WOMEN

What about the older population, particularly women who have reached menopause? Menopause is a pivotal moment in bone health, because at this point, levels of estrogen suddenly fall. Normally, estrogen helps to maintain bone mass by switching off the processes that tend to break down bone. So menopause is crucial, a tipping point after which bone mineral content often falls quite rapidly, as shown in the earlier figure.

Again, however, the news is good for those who are regular runners or wish to start exercise. Regular exercise helps increase BMC slightly during this time, when the norm is for the mineral content to fall relatively rapidly. For example, Gail Dalsky of the University of Connecticut had a group of postmenopausal women do quite high-intensity exercise, including running up and down concrete stairs, and found that the BMC of the spine increased by 5.2 percent. The inactive controls experienced a decline of 1.4 percent over the same 9-month period, which means exercise produced a 6.6 percent swing over inactivity in less than a year. This is a pretty big difference, much larger than many other studies have found, and is probably the result of a combination of factors. Exercise is one of them, but many of the women in this study were also on hormone-replacement therapy. We won't discuss hormone therapy in detail here, other than to say that the evidence suggests that if you combine exercise with hormone therapy, you tend to gain more bone mass than if you use either alone. So even if you are on hormone therapy, there is scope for greater improvement through exercise.

There is also a very specific effect on different bones, depending on the exercise performed. You can target the spine, the hip, or the femur by doing different kinds of exercise. For example, targeted loading of the spine is done using high-impact running (like the concrete stair study described previously) and weight training. The femur and hip are loaded substantially more during walking, running, and rowing, though there is substantial crossover, and weight training can be used to target any bone group. The practical implication is that an all-round exercise program, consisting of some high-impact activity such as running, some low-impact activity such as walking, and a whole-body weight-training program, will provide the best overall result for the whole skeleton.

The high-impact aspect of exercise seems to provide the biggest benefit, which of course presents us with a dilemma. Often, postmenopausal women who begin exercise training have been inactive for many years and have relatively weak bones (as well as weak muscles, tendons, and cardiovascular systems). These women are very susceptible to overuse injuries, so great care must be taken to avoid overdoing early exercise. The key principle of overload applies—one should find the exact volume and intensity of training that stresses the bone just enough to cause adaptation and then plan a long-term training program, instead of blindly following a guideline that says that high-impact exercise is best. Once again, with exercise you need to be in it for the long haul, so be patient and work toward improving your body's ability to handle that exercise.

MEN

We hope men don't feel left out of the discussion, since we've devoted a couple of pages to pre- and postmenopausal women. The same principles apply to you. In fact, osteoporosis is being increasingly recognized as a problem among men. It's not as bad, because peak bone mass in men is greater than in women, the decline is usually less—5 percent per decade compared with 10 percent in women—and men don't have the menopause factor. However, that doesn't mean that men should not be concerned about osteoporosis, weak bones, and fractures, particularly later in life.

Men's bones respond pretty much the same as women's bones to exercise and to running in particular, with a small increase in mineral density brought about by weight training or impact exercises. Again, the value is not only in the short-term increase but in the fact that exercise prevents the aging-related decline that affects inactive people.

PEOPLE WITH OSTEOPOROSIS

The final group to consider is people who have already developed osteoporosis. This condition profoundly increases the risk of fracture, because the bone is so weakened by the decline in mineral content that it often fractures under the smallest load. Exercise would seem to be a risk for these individuals, but properly managed training has been found to improve bone health even in this group. The trick, of course, is the management of exercise, along with other treatment methods. Exercise is probably not the most effective form of treatment—that distinction goes to therapies including estrogen and progesterone. But exercise is vital because it also improves muscle strength, balance, coordination, and general well-being, which reduce risk of falling in the first place. (Elderly women without osteoporosis are typically 20 percent stronger than women with osteoporosis.)

The bottom line is that exercise works. In men and women, young and old, strong or weak, impact exercises such as running increase bone mass and prevent its decline. However, the trick is to understand that prescribing exercise is much like prescribing medication—there is an optimal dose, and too little will not work, while too much can be disastrous. It's therefore vital that you get the balance right. There are no hard-and-fast rules, however, because each person is unique. If you have years of running behind you, the advice is "more of the same." If you are older and inspired to take up running, you will have to begin with something like walking, so that you don't push your body too hard, too soon. The addition of weight training is especially valuable because it allows targeting of specific bones, which running does not. A balanced program, particularly later in life, is crucial to optimum bone health.

The Influence of Diet on Bone—Drink Your Milk for Healthy Bones?

Finally, diet is a key factor that contributes to bone strength, because calcium is such an integral part of bone. It's not alone, though—vitamin D is the other nutrient that plays a really important role in the development of a strong skeleton.

The role of calcium is particularly well known, and a huge industry has sprung up around calcium supplementation in particular (see above). The theory is that calcium in high doses at any stage of life, will help to prevent conditions such as osteoporosis from developing. The theoretical basis seems sound enough, but the evidence does not clearly support this theory. This is partly because your body begins to retain less calcium as a result of low calcium levels. Scientists call this phenomenon calcium retention efficiency, and it basically says that as you take in more and more calcium, your body retains less and less of it, the result being that your bone retention of calcium is relatively unaffected by megadoses. By the same theory, people who take in very little calcium per day might still have healthy bones thanks to greater retention.

Another key factor is that when you look at people who are incorporating high amounts of calcium in their diets, they often do so as a result of high overall energy intakes. We know that high nutrient intakes tend to be found in people who do regular exercise, and that nutrient-deficient diets are detrimental to bone mass. We are therefore easily misled into thinking that it is the calcium that is responsible, when in fact it is the physical activity level and overall nutrient intake that are responsible.

Adequate vitamin D is also vital for bone health because when this vitamin is deficient, the body secretes hormones that ultimately increase the breakdown of bone and reduce BMC. The body makes vitamin D on its own when skin is exposed to sunlight, and because most of us runners are outdoors in sunlight indulging in our exercise habit, we're unlikely to be deficient in this vitamin. Vitamin D is not naturally abundant in food but has become more widely available, as most countries now add vitamin D to dairy products. Even so, recent evidence suggests that vitamin D deficiency is more widespread and causing more health problems than previously thought. A recent study from Harvard Medical School estimated that 30 to 40 percent of Americans are vitamin D deficient. Many experts believe that it is not possible to maintain adequate vitamin D levels without frequent exposure to sunlight.

Finally, when you think about nutrition for bone health, you probably don't think of fruits and vegetables, but a number of studies

Calcium Supplementation?

Studies have failed to find an effect of calcium supplementation on bone mass or mineral content in premenopausal years. During the early postmenopausal years, BMC decreases rapidly as a result of the removal of the ovarian hormones (estrogen and progesterone), and calcium supplementation does little to prevent this process. Supplementation is believed, however, to prevent bone loss of just under 1 percent per year if taken in very high doses (about 1 gram per day). In the later postmenopausal years, when the risk of osteoporosis is higher, calcium seems to prevent bone loss, helping women maintain their bone mass.

Certain types of calcium are more effective than others. Soluble calcium salts and dairy products are best, whereas calcium carbonate is ineffective. Also, a lot depends on calcium intake before supplementation. If it was low, the supplemental calcium is more effective. But if prior calcium intake was above roughly 400 milligrams per day, supplementation has little or no effect.

So if you're concerned about calcium intake, perhaps as a result of restricted dairy intake, then calcium supplements can prove useful, particularly later in life. However, dietary calcium is preferred, and most people should get their daily intake from their diets. Also, a combination of other factors, including exercise and healthy lifestyle (not smoking, for example), is likely to be more effective than adequate calcium intake alone in preventing a decrease in BMC during the earlier years of life.

have demonstrated a strong link between higher rates of fruit and vegetable consumption and better bone health. Why? In part it's because fruits and vegetables help the body maintain its natural pH balance. When metabolized, fruits and vegetables produce natural buffers that neutralize the acids produced by meats and grains. When there aren't a lot of fruits and vegetables in the diet, the body must resort to pulling minerals from the bones to achieve this buffering effect. But in people who eat plenty of fresh fruits and vegetables, bone minerals are allowed to stay where they belong—in the bones.

Chapter 4

Weak in the Knees

Distance running has a higher injury rate than most other sports. Consider the results of a recent Dutch study, in which more than 700 participants in the Rotterdam Marathon were surveyed about injuries suffered during the process of training for the event and within the marathon itself. Nearly 55 percent of the respondents reported suffering at least one running-related leg injury within the preceding year, and 18 percent developed an injury during the marathon itself.

Other studies of running injuries have generated results supporting the same general conclusion—running is hard on the human musculoskeletal system. Another Dutch study tracked injuries in a group of 629 recreational runners training for a four-mile event. In just eight weeks, nearly 26 percent of these runners developed at least one injury.

Why is running so hard on the muscles, bones, and connective tissues? One factor is repetition. The vast majority of running injuries are classified as overuse injuries, meaning they develop slowly with repeated stress on certain tissues, causing them to degenerate. When running, you take 70 to 90 strides per leg per minute. If you run an hour a day Tuesday through Sunday, you're repeating the stride motion nearly 30,000 times per week. There are a lot of movements besides running that would cause body tissues to wear out if you repeated them that often.

Yet competitive swimmers repeat swim strokes with comparable frequency, and many competitive cyclists complete many more pedal strokes each week than runners do strides, but the injury rates in swimming and cycling are significantly lower than those in running. This unfortunate difference was pointed out in a 1998 study involving triathletes, who, of course, do a lot of swimming, cycling, and running. Researchers at Straffordshire University in England found that among elite triathletes, 62.1 percent of injuries suffered during a five-year period were caused by running, 34.5 percent by cycling, and only 3.4 percent by swimming. Among midlevel triathletes, the numbers were 64.3 percent, 25.0 percent, and 10.7 percent. Among recreational triathletes, percentages shifted a bit toward swimming, with a breakdown of 58.7 percent running injuries, 15.9 percent cycling injuries, and 15.4 percent swimming injuries.

The key difference between running and the other triathlon disciplines is impact: Running is a high-impact activity, whereas swimming and cycling produce no impact. So clearly it's repetitive *impact* rather than repetition *per se* that makes the injury rate in running so high compared with other sports.

Each time your foot makes contact with the ground, forces equaling two to four times your body weight travel upward through your lower leg, knee, thigh, hip, and pelvis, and into your spine. These forces rattle the tissues of your lower body in much the same way the seismic forces of an earthquake rattle the walls of buildings. But just as some buildings remain standing through an earthquake while others fall, impact forces from running do not equally disrupt all the tissues they pass through. Instead, damage is concentrated in areas of greater susceptibility.

These areas differ from runner to runner

and even within the same runner over time. Newer runners are more likely to suffer tibial bone strains, or tissue degeneration in the larger of the two lower-leg bones. Remember that with repeated stress and recovery, bone adapts by becoming denser and stiffer, thus more injury-resistant; novice runners have not yet achieved the adaptations that take many months and perhaps years of consistent running to develop. Faster runners and those who do more high-speed training, on the other hand, are more likely to develop Achilles tendinosis, or tissue degeneration in the Achilles tendon, because strain on this tendon increases dramatically with increasing running speed. Pronounced heel-strikers are more likely to develop patellofemoral pain syndrome (PFPS), or tissue degeneration under the kneecap, because impact forces are transferred more abruptly from the foot to the knee in such runners. Finally, women are much more likely than men to develop PFPS and tibial stress fractures, due to anatomical differences in their body structure.

Given these observations and your obvious desire to avoid becoming one of the perhaps 60 percent of runners who will become injured, you are no doubt wondering how you might go about preventing injury. There are three general ways to reduce the likelihood that such breakdowns will occur: running less, reducing the impact force and its effects on susceptible tissues, and increasing the resilience of the tissues of the lower extremities.

Running Less

We've all heard the following joke: A man goes to a doctor and says, "Doc, it hurts when I lift my arm." So the doctor says, "Well, then, don't lift your arm!" The same logic applies to running. The most obvious way to minimize the risk of suffering running-related injuries is to limit the frequency of stride repetitions (in other words, to limit your running mileage) to a level that is beneath the threshold for degeneration in your most susceptible areas. This threshold is different for individual runners, and it changes over time for any single runner. The trouble with limiting running mileage as a strategy to reduce injury risk, however, is that increasing running mileage is one of the most effective ways to improve running fitness and performance. So while it's important that you run fewer miles than the number that puts you at high risk of injury, for the sake of optimizing your performance, you also want to run as much mileage as possible without crossing that threshold. You are on a tightrope between insufficient training to improve and excessive training that breaks you down.

The only way to know where this threshold lies is to cross it unwittingly once in a while and become injured or develop symptoms of an incipient injury. Through such experience, you will develop a better feel for your body's limits, which will enable you to remain more often on the safe side of the injury threshold. Finding the right balance between running enough to build fitness and running infrequently enough to stay healthy is a matter of gradually increasing your training load according to a sensible plan, backing off whenever a sore spot warns of a potential breakdown, and never running more than necessary to achieve your goals.

Reducing Impact and Its Effects

A second way to reduce the likelihood of injury is to either reduce the amount of impact force that your body is subjected to or disperse impact forces so that they don't concentrate as heavily in your most susceptible tissues. This can be done to a small degree by switching to shoes that reduce the amount of impact forces the body absorbs (through different cushioning characteristics) or to shoes that better disperse impact forces (through different stability characteristics). Switching from harder running surfaces such as asphalt to softer surfaces such as grass also has a small effect on impact forces. Running in shallow or deep water or on an antigravity treadmill or an elliptical trainer is a more drastic approach to reducing impact forces. Because these alternatives are less practical (antigravity treadmills are very hard to find and cost $75,000) and, for most runners, less enjoyable than normal running, they are most often resorted to only by runners who have an injury that prevents them from running but does not prevent them from engaging in similar low- or nonimpact activities. However, these options can be routinely used for injury prevention as well.

There is some evidence that altering one's running form and strengthening certain muscles may reduce the degree to which impact forces concentrate in particular areas, causing tissue degeneration. For example, Irene Davis, PhD, of the University of Delaware, conducted a study in which she trained a small group of runners suffering from PFPS to prevent their thighs from rotating internally during the stance phase of the stride. Previous research had established a link between this form abnormality, which results from weak hip abductor and external rotator muscles, and PFPS. After eight gait-retraining sessions performed on a treadmill in a four-week period, knee pain had diminished in all subjects to zero from a starting point of 5 to 7 points on a 10-point scale. This study was not controlled (in other words, there were no injured runners who kept running in their natural way for comparison's sake), but the results are noteworthy nevertheless.

Research into the effects of targeted strength training on the risk of specific running injuries is as nascent as research on gait retraining. In some of the earliest research in this area, Swedish scientists found that eccentric calf muscle strengthening exercises such as the eccentric heel dip (see page 60) were a very effective treatment for Achilles tendinosis in runners. More recently, research by Paul Niemuth, of the University of St. Catherine in Minnesota, suggested that strengthening exercises for the hip abductors and hip external rotators may reduce the risk of PFPS and iliotibial band syndrome.

Another leading researcher in the area of muscle strength and running injuries is Michael Fredericson, MD, of Stanford University. Although he has not established a scientifically rigorous connection between weakness in the abdominal musculature and running injuries, his extensive clinical experience tells him that the relationship definitely exists. Dr. Fredericson created a comprehensive core-strength training program for runners, which includes exercises such as the side bridge (see page 58). It's an extremely well-designed program, and we highly recommend that any interested runner follow the whole program. You can find it online at solpt.com/images/Coretraining.pdf.

Developing More Resilient Legs

Increasing the resilience of the tissues most susceptible to impact forces and their effects also reduces the likelihood of developing overuse injuries. Through proper training, you can greatly enhance the durability of your bones, muscles, and connective tissues and thereby significantly increase the amount of running you can do before breaking down. For the competitive runner who wishes to train as hard as necessary to achieve his or her goals without becoming injured, improving the durability of tissues is without

(continued on page 61)

Strength Exercises for Injury Prevention

Performing the following strength exercise three times per week may reduce your risk of developing certain overuse injuries.

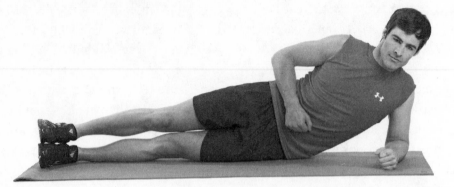

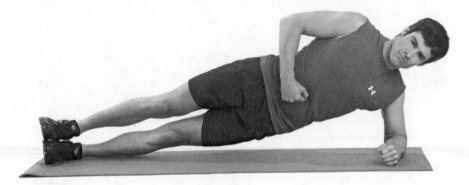

Side Bridge
STRENGTHENS THE LUMBAR STABILIZERS, IMPROVING PELVIC AND SPINAL STABILITY

Lie on your right side with your legs fully extended and stacked and your right arm bent 90 degrees, with your forearm on the floor. Lift your hips until your body forms a straight line from neck to ankles. You may want to do this exercise in front of a mirror to make sure your hips don't sag toward the floor. Hold the bridge position for 20 to 30 seconds and then flip over and repeat. Alternate sides for the desired number of repetitions.

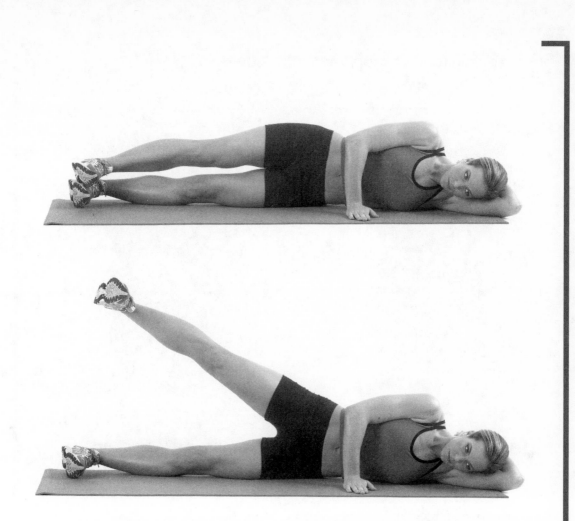

Side-Lying Leg Raise
CONDITIONS THE HIP ABDUCTORS AND HIP EXTERNAL ROTATORS, ENHANCING HIP STABILITY AND REDUCING THE RISK OF PFPS AND ILIOTIBIAL BAND SYNDROME

Lie on your side with your legs extended and stacked. Repeatedly lift the top leg toward the ceiling (toes pointing forward) as high as you can. Repeat the movement 12 to 15 times and then switch sides. To make this exercise more challenging, do it with an ankle weight strapped to the ankle of your working leg.

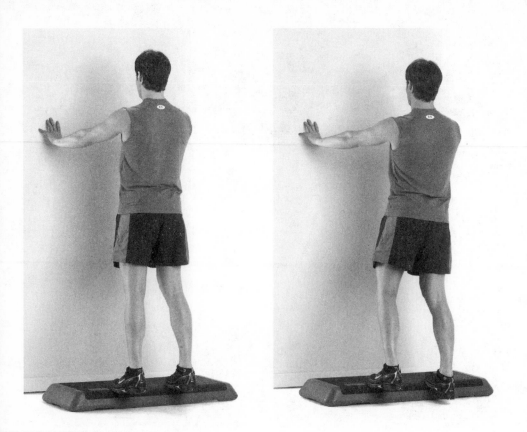

Eccentric Heel Dip
**STRENGTHENS THE CALF MUSCLE–ACHILLES TENDON COMPLEX,
REDUCING THE RISK OF ACHILLES TENDINOSIS**

Balance on one foot on a sturdy platform or step, with the ball of the foot resting on the edge of the platform so that the unsupported heel hangs over the back of the platform. Rest your fingertips against a wall or some other support for balance. Lower your heel toward the floor until you feel a stretch in your calf muscles—your heel will drop below the level of the ball of your foot. Then raise your heel to a neutral position. At first, when you lift your heel to the starting position, do so using both legs to avoid overloading the calf muscle. Once it's stronger, you may attempt the lifting phase using one calf. Always use one calf for the lowering phase. Do 8 to 16 repetitions and then switch feet.

question the most important way to prevent injuries. Let's take a much closer look at this approach to injury prevention.

USE IT (BUT DON'T OVERUSE IT) OR LOSE IT

In 2002, Michael Muller, a professor of physical therapy at Washington University, presented a new theory of tissue adaptation to physical stress that provides a helpful conceptual framework for runners seeking to stay healthy without sacrificing performance. Physical stress theory, as it is called, is essentially an adaptation of Selye's General Adaptation Principle, which you will recall from the Introduction. Muller's theory is based specifically on the simple premise that body tissues adapt in a predictable way in response to changes in the relative level of physical stress they are exposed to. When tissues are exposed to an accustomed level of stress, they maintain their current structure and function—a state that is often referred to as homeostasis. When these same tissues are exposed to a slight or gradual increase in stress, they modify their structure and function—after an initial period of breakdown (recall the muscle damage and the "morning-after problem" of Chapter 2)—to become more tolerant of that type of stress. They achieve a new homeostasis at an increased level of durability.

For example, a recent animal study found that when rats were exposed to a running program, fingerlike branches of new tissue grew in the attachments between the tendons and muscles of their legs, strengthening these important junctions. But if a stress is increased too quickly or abruptly, the tissues never recover from the initial period of breakdown. They lose their homeostatic balance and progressively degenerate. All running overuse injuries follow this pattern.

On the other hand, if the level of stress is reduced, the tissues adapt in the other direction, finding a new homeostasis at a lower level of durability and function. This is why (to choose an extreme example) astronauts lose significant amounts of bone mass, muscle mass, and even blood volume without the accustomed stress of gravity to resist. Their situation becomes so dire that upon returning to the gravitational force of the earth's surface they often struggle to stand upright, so weak are their muscles, joints, and bones. It takes time for them to "relearn" these basic functions, illustrating how remarkably adaptable your body is, as captured in Muller's physical stress model.

The physical stress theory reminds us that running does not only cause overuse injuries—it also protects us against them. When you increase your running volume at a sensible rate and then maintain your mileage at a sensible upper limit, the tissues of your lower body become significantly better able to tolerate the stress of running, without losing homeostasis.

Perhaps the most basic example is that of bone density. Runners have greater bone density in their legs than nonrunners, as a consequence of the adaptive response of bone tissue to the repetitive impact of running. Consequently, a trained runner who goes for a run of any given distance will experience less bone tissue damage than a nonrunner who runs an equal distance. And there's some evidence that a moderate- or high-mileage runner will experience less bone damage than a low-mileage runner; one study found that higher-mileage runners had greater bone density than their lower-mileage counterparts (who in turn had greater bone density than nonrunners).

Several studies have demonstrated that experienced runners who have been training for several years are significantly less likely to become injured than beginning runners. While this may be the case in part because some of the most injury-prone novice runners quit, leaving fewer injury-prone runners to become more experienced, it is undoubtedly also a result of the durability-increasing tissue adaptations that more experienced runners have earned. Another factor is the much greater relative increases in physical stress that beginners typically experience relative to veteran runners. The bones, muscles, and joint tissues of the person who's going from zero to 20 miles a week in training for his or her first 5-K are more likely to lose their homeostatic balance than those of a veteran runner who's

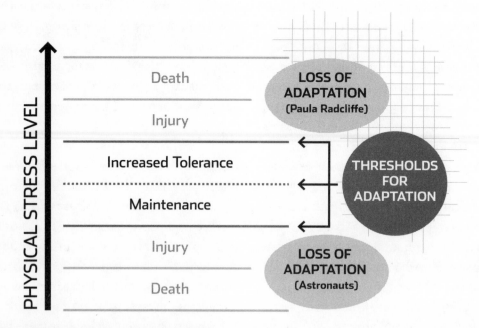

Effect of Physical Stress on Tissue Adaptation
This table graphically summarizes Michael Muller's physical stress theory, which is important for every runner to understand.

training from 40 to 60 miles per week to set a 10-K personal record (PR).

On the other hand, the single best predictor of running injuries is running mileage. Those who run the most miles per week have the highest risk of injury. To be sure, thanks to the greater durability of their lower-body tissues, high-mileage runners typically experience far fewer injuries per hour spent running than low-mileage runners do, but because they spend so much more time running, they experience more injuries on a yearly basis. It seems to be a Catch-22: You need to run more to increase the injury resistance of your legs, but the relative increase in physical stress that comes with running more often exceeds the resulting increase in durability, so you wind up with injuries more often.

It may be possible, however, to get the fitness and durability benefits of running more miles without increasing your injury risk to the degree that high mileage does. Just follow these three guidelines:

Ramp up slowly. As the physical stress theory shows, whether an increase in physical stress makes a tissue stronger or breaks it down is determined by the magnitude of that increase. In running, this translates to the rate at which you increase your weekly mileage. By ramping up very slowly—the often-cited rule is 10 percent per week (though some people have to limit it to 5 percent, while others can make much larger increases)—you expose your leg tissues to manageable amounts of damage that can be repaired and adapted to before the next run. When your tissues are given the opportunity to fully restore their prior homeostasis between runs, then, by definition, you *can't* get injured—by definition—because an injury is a loss of homeostasis.

Obey your pain. Interestingly, a study involving novice runners found that those who ramped up according to the 10 percent rule suffered just as many injuries as those who jumped into a steady level of training. So, clearly, the advice to "ramp up slowly" is not sufficient in itself to reduce injury risk—at least in beginners. But we're willing to bet that the runners in this study would have broken down less often if they had complemented the 10 percent rule with a second guideline: When something starts to hurt, run less.

No numerical rule can predict how your body will respond to your training. While, in the long run, using the 10 percent rule will certainly keep you healthier than if you included abrupt mileage spikes in your training, it still doesn't make any sense to continue increasing your running mileage at a rate of 10 percent per week if you've developed a sore spot that gets a little worse every time you run. You must never ignore pain. This is so important that we will repeat it: *Do not ignore pain.* When you develop a sore spot, reduce your running just enough to make the pain go away, and then begin increasing your mileage cautiously. Sometimes it's necessary to stop running completely for a few days, but that is more than worth it when you consider that the possible consequences of ignoring the pain and continuing to run might be many weeks off later with a far more serious injury.

Be consistent. Research suggests that injuries are more likely to occur during periods of increasing running mileage than they are during periods of steady mileage, even if that steady mileage level is high. According to the physical stress model, simple repetition of a familiar stress is unlikely to cause a loss of homeostasis, which in running means that you're unlikely to break down when maintaining your mileage at a consistently high level after you've safely brought it up to that high level.

Naturally, high mileage is relative. As a general rule, avoid letting your weekly mileage dip below 50 percent of your peak weekly mileage. So if your heaviest training week during the year is 50 miles, try to avoid running fewer than 25 miles at any other time of the year, except perhaps during a brief (one- or two-week) off-season break.

Training Intensity: The Often-Forgotten Variable

One final factor, implied when we spoke about ramping up your training mileage slowly, is that intensity, or running speed, is just as important a predictor of running injuries or adaptation as mileage is. In our experience, it may be even more vital. The most dangerous period for many runners is that moment when they decide they have reached a plateau of weekly volume and are going to introduce weekly speedwork sessions or time trials or races into their program.

A sudden addition of higher-speed running increases the relative impact per session by an exponential amount. If the overall running volume is not reduced in line with the increase in running intensity, the combined effect is the same as if you massively increased your distance. It's vital to appreciate that it's not simply repetition but repetition of impact that precipitates injuries; thus both intensity and impact must be managed in the same way as volume—small increases, gradual adaptation, and consistency.

The bottom line is this: Smart training is the most effective way to balance your goals of maximizing running performance and minimizing injury risk. Wearing the right shoes, improving your running form, and strengthening your key stabilizing muscles are helpful secondary measures to increase the amount of running you can do without breaking down.

The Big Five

The five most common overuse injuries in runners are patellofemoral pain syndrome, iliotibial band syndrome, plantar fasciitis, tibial bone strains, and Achilles tendinosis. Information follows, based on the latest research, about the nature of each injury and how to prevent and overcome it.

PATELLOFEMORAL PAIN SYNDROME (PFPS)

Patellofemoral pain syndrome, otherwise known as anterior knee pain and runner's knee, is the most common running injury, accounting for roughly 20 percent of all running injuries.

Description and Causes

The main symptom is pain under the kneecap. Pain is generally mild at first and experienced only during running, but it becomes progressively more intense during running and is also increasingly felt at rest if training continues.

Many theories about the nature of the damage underlying the pain have come and gone. The reason behind this revolving door of proposed etiologies is that, unlike other injuries such as knee meniscus damage, there is no obvious structural abnormality associated with PFPS, whether the joint is examined by X-ray, MRI, or surgical arthroscope. Recently this conundrum has led orthopedists to formulate a new view of PFPS, in which pain itself—more specifically, chronic stimulation of pain nerves in the knee—is understood as the essence of the injury. Relatively minor degradation in any of a number of knee tissues, such as inflammation of the synovium, a pouch that contains the knee's lubricating fluid, may underlie this pain nerve stimulation. But because these breakdowns are relatively minor and hard to identify, they need not be targeted. The pain itself must be targeted.

Training through It

How do you target the pain? First, you avoid doing anything, including running, that causes the knee to hurt, but you also do as much pain-free running as you can do. This approach will enable the damaged tissues to restore homeostasis (their natural equilibrium state of breakdown and regeneration) while also keeping the knee well adapted to the stress of running. Many runners with PFPS can do some pain-free running. You might find that you can run for a certain duration (say, 20 minutes)—and no longer—without pain. In this case, run only that distance until your limit increases. You might find that you can run every other day, but not every day, without pain. In this case, run every other day for a while. After a few weeks, try a test run 24 hours after a previous run to see whether the limit remains. Continue to gradually increase your running toward pre-injury levels as comfort allows, reversing this process briefly whenever soreness emerges anew.

Treatment and Rehabilitation

Where there is pain, there is almost always inflammation. Taking a nonsteroidal anti-inflammatory medication (NSAID) such as ibuprofen according to label directions and placing an ice pack on your knee for 10 minutes at a time, three times a day, may accelerate the resolution of the inflammation.

Consider whether poor shoe selection, biomechanical factors, and/or muscle weakness might have contributed to your injury. Weakness in the hip abductors and hip external rotators is often seen in PFPS sufferers. In runners whose hip stabilizers are weak, the thigh tends to rotate internally as the foot comes in contact with the ground. This is a compensatory movement, performed unconsciously to enable other muscles to take up the job of stabilizing the pelvis. But these other muscles can't entirely take up the slack, and consequently the pelvis tilts laterally toward the ground on the side of the unsupported leg. The thigh tilts with it, like a falling tower, while the lower leg remains upright, pinching the knee between them. This pinching effect, along with the twisted (or "knock-kneed") position of the thigh relative to the knee when it absorbs impact forces, causes damage within the joint. If you are a knock-kneed runner, train yourself to actively contract the muscles on the outside of your hips when you run to keep your pelvis level and maintain your thighs in their natural, neutral alignment. As mentioned previously, Irene Davis successfully taught a group of PFPS sufferers to control this movement by strengthening and activating the relevant muscle groups. In addition, begin doing exercises such as the side lying leg raise (see page 59) to strengthen the hip abductors and hip external rotators.

It is possible that pronounced heel striking, or overstriding, also increases the risk for PFPS. While this link has not been shown directly, studies have demonstrated that runners who experience excessive impact shock are more likely to develop PFPS and that heel strikers experience greater impact shock than knock-kneed runners. If you are a pronounced heelstriker and you have PFPS, train yourself to shorten your stride and land with your foot flat underneath your hips instead of heel-first out in front of your body.

If reducing impact shock is an effective means of reducing the risk of PFPS, then switching to running shoes that reduce impact shock may also protect the knees. The problem is that research on the relationship between shoe cushioning and impact shock has produced muddled results. Some studies have found that impact forces are actually greater in running shoes with softer cushioning, due to unconscious stride changes that are made in different shoes. However, it has been suggested that such counterintuitive results may result from inadequate measurement techniques. At least one recent study provides evidence that added shoe cushioning reduces specific impact variables that are now understood as the best indicators of injury risk—namely, peak loading rate (the abruptness of impact) and tibial acceleration rate (the rate at which the lower leg approaches the ground).

However, it still seems to be true that interaction between the specific shoe and the individual runner has a major effect on impact characteristics; the right level of cushioning is different for each runner, and it's impossible to predict the level that is right for any single runner.

Since you can't undergo comprehensive impact testing when shopping for running shoes, how do you select the shoe with the right amount of cushioning to minimize your risk of developing PFPS and other injuries? Some research indicates that comfort is a fairly reliable guide. Subjective assessments of comfort coupled with on-the-road experience are even better. To begin, buy and wear the most comfortable shoe you can find. If it keeps you injury-free, buy another pair (or buy the most similar pair you can find when that particular model is inevitably phased out or replaced with a newer version). If you become injured in that shoe, try a different shoe that is also very comfortable with a little more or less cushioning. Keep experimenting with different shoes until you find your optimal shoe type (Keep in mind that even the optimal shoe will not prevent all injuries if training volume, intensity, and increases are not smartly managed, as described).

The good news about patellofemoral pain syndrome is that it's a relatively minor condition, a chronic failure of tissues within the knee to recover fully from normal running-induced damage between runs. The bad news is that it can be just as debilitating and last just as long as more serious breakdowns. Use the tips we've just given you to minimize the impact (so to speak) of knee pain on your running, if and when it strikes.

ILIOTIBIAL BAND SYNDROME (ITBS)

Iliotibial band syndrome is the second-most-common running injury after PFPS.

Description and Causes

The IT band is a long band of tendinous tissue that originates on the outside of the pelvis and runs along the outer thigh all the way past the knee, attaching to the tibia. It provides lateral support for the leg, helping to prevent the pelvis from tipping to the side when only one foot is in contact with the ground. It has been proposed that during running, the IT band passes from behind the femur to the front side of the femur as the hip extends. As this happens, the lower part of the IT band may rub against the bulbous end of the femur, causing friction. As the stride is repeated thousands upon thousands of times, the constant friction causes tissue breakdown, inflammation, and thickening of the band in this area. Pain emerges at the knee or ankle and becomes increasingly intense and long-lasting as training continues. Less commonly, pain occurs just below the hip.

Recently the traditional explanation of ITBS has been challenged. Welsh researchers have noted that the IT band is not a discrete structure capable of sliding back and forth along the thigh but is instead essentially "glued" to the thigh musculature, making friction against the lower femur impossible. They have proposed that the injury actually results from compression of a layer of fat and loose connective tissue situated between the IT band and the lower femur. We'll let the anatomy experts squabble over this one—it makes little difference in terms of how you treat and prevent the problem.

Weak hip stabilizers elevate the risk of ITBS by increasing tension on the IT band during the ground contact phase of the stride. The internal rotation of the thigh, which goes hand-in-hand with hip weakness, frequently causes PFPS, and is commonly apparent in ITBS sufferers, further strains the IT band. So the same strength exercises and gait modifications that overcome PFPS may help you beat ITBS as well.

Treatment and Rehabilitation

Michael Fredericson, the Stanford University running injury expert mentioned earlier, conducted a study that provided evidence of the effectiveness of strengthening of the hip stabilizers. He put 24 runners with ITBS through a six-week standard rehabilitation program supplemented with strength training. At the end of it, all of the runners were pain-free, and after six months, 22 of the 24 remained healthy. This study had no control, so we don't know how well the runners would have done without strength training, but 22 out of 24 is not bad!

You can use the usual inflammation controls—icing and anti-inflammatory medication—to treat the symptoms of ITBS, but don't expect to need much pain relief if you reduce your running sufficiently. Sports massage, on the other hand, often provides a measure of immediate relief to runners with this particular injury. Deep tissue work on a damaged IT band can be extremely painful, but it lengthens the IT band just enough to reduce friction (or compression) and enable the runner to do some training as the rehabilitation process continues. As an alternative or complement to professional sports massage, you may also benefit from self-massage using a therapeutic foam roller. Lie on your right side, with the foam roller beneath the outside of your upper thigh and your arms supporting your torso. Use your arms to pull yourself forward so that your thigh slides over the roller from just below the hip to just above the knee. Put as much weight on your IT band as it can tolerate. Roll back and forth several times and then switch sides.

There is no clear relationship between footwear and ITBS. As with all injuries, you should consider inappropriate footwear as a possible contributing factor to your ITBS. Try to find a more comfortable shoe if you determine that your current shoe might be at least partly to blame. A more likely contributor to your breakdown is running too many laps in the same direction on the track, a mistake that may lead to a left-right strength imbalance in the hips. Similarly, running on cambered roads places different stress on the inside as opposed to the outside leg, which

Does Overpronation Really Cause Running Injuries?

For many years, experts on running injuries believed—and taught—that overpronation (an excessive inward roll) of the foot during the stance phase of running causes a large percentage of the overuse injuries that runners experience. As a result, running shoe manufacturers have developed all manner of antipronation features for their footwear, and podiatrists have made a killing by prescribing antipronation orthotic shoe inserts. But there's actually very little evidence that a high degree of pronation increases the risk of any specific type of injury. A few scattered studies have found correlations, but for each such study, there's another with results that contradict it. And it's worth noting that in many cases taking off your shoes and running barefoot will actually reduce overpronation more than switching to more rigid (some would say "overbuilt") shoes.

The jury is out on this one. Our advice is to focus on managing the crucial aspects, those known to cause injuries, such as your training volume, intensity, muscle strength factors, and methods to reduce impact, as we've described in this chapter.

can result in the same problem. Overcoming this issue is simply a matter of providing variety, which balances out the impact stresses and minimizes injury risk.

Interestingly, fast running tends to be less problematic for ITBS sufferers than slower running. Therefore you might want to initiate your return to normal training by supplementing your cross-training workouts with a few relaxed sprints to maintain as much of your running-specific fitness adaptation as possible while you recover.

PLANTAR FASCIITIS

Plantar fasciitis is one of the more difficult injuries to shake. The location of the injury on the underside of the foot makes reducing tissue stress enough to allow the damaged tissues to restore homeostasis a challenge. Some cases persist for years, and none of us wants that.

Description and Causes

The plantar fascia is a tough web of tissue on the underside of the foot that supports the structural integrity of the arch. When the foot impacts the ground during running, the plantar fascia stretches to allow the foot to flatten and roll and then retracts to its normal length by force of its internal tension as the foot leaves the ground. This repetitive stretching against tension may strain the tissue of the plantar fascia that lies close to its attachment point in the heel bone. As damage accumulates, inflammation sets in and pain emerges.

Training through It

If you catch the problem early enough, you may be able to overcome it with a moderate reduction in running mileage. However, if it becomes severe, you may have to stop running altogether for a few weeks. Let pain be your guide—never run beyond the point of moderate discomfort. Cross-train in modalities that you can do pain-free to maintain fitness and reduce the temptation to resume normal running training too quickly.

Treatment and Rehabilitation

The more aggressive treatments for plantar fasciitis—namely cortisone injections and shock wave therapy—work best, but most physicians are reluctant to prescribe them for those who have had the injury for less than six months. If you can't shake your heel pain in a few weeks, push for the more aggressive treatments, which elite runners routinely get early.

One of the reasons plantar fasciitis often takes so long to heal is that most of the healing occurs at night, when the fascia is relaxed. Once you wake up and put weight on your foot, it stretches out, and eight hours' worth of healing is undone in an instant. Wearing a night splint may accelerate the healing of your damaged fascia by limiting the setback that comes with standing for the first time each morning. Stretching your plantar fascia before you get out of bed in the morning and after any long period of sitting may further accelerate your recovery by limiting the small

amount of injury you incur during the day when you put your full body weight on your feet. Benedict DiGiovanni of the University of Rochester developed the following stretch for plantar fasciitis sufferers: In a sitting position, cross your injured-side leg over the other leg and use your hands to hyperextend your toes for 10 seconds. Relax and repeat the stretch a total of 10 times. In a study of this treatment, 75 percent of patients were pain-free and able to do their normal activities within three to six months, and only 25 percent required any further treatment.

Poor ankle flexibility is a significant risk factor for plantar fasciitis. To improve your ankle flexibility, try this exercise: Stand facing a wall, with the toes of one foot against the wall, and bend the knee forward to tap the wall with your kneecap. Now slide the foot back a bit so that your toes are about an inch away from the wall, and repeat. Keep moving back little by little until you get to the point where the kneecap is *barely* touching the wall. Make sure that your knee aims straight forward and not inward (knock-kneed) and that the heel remains on the floor the entire time. Perform eight repetitions with each leg.

Podiatrists and physical therapists often recommend motion control running shoes and orthotic shoe inserts for plantar fasciitis suffers. These changes are intended to reduce foot pronation during running, which is widely believed to contribute to the condition. However, there is little scientific evidence that overpronation contributes to plantar fasciitis. That said, finding a more comfortable running shoe—specifically one that reduces heel pain—may well help you overcome the injury more quickly and reduce the risk of recurrence. If that's a more stable shoe (or an orthotic insert), so be it, but be open-minded in your search.

TIBIAL BONE STRAINS

The bones of the lower leg, especially the tibia, which is the more delicate of the two, are among the most injury-susceptible tissues in beginning runners (and those beginning anew after a layoff). Injuries in this area occur far more commonly in beginning runners than in experienced ones. Injuries in the bones of the lower leg were previously lumped together under one diagnosis—"shinsplints"—but it's now been recognized that shinsplints is not necessarily a diagnosis but rather a symptom of one of many potential injuries that affect the tibia.

Description and Causes

Bone tissue is continuously dismantled and rebuilt in runners and nonrunners alike. When you start a running program, this two-step remodeling process accelerates. First, existing bone tissue is dismantled. Next, new, denser, stronger bone tissue is formed. But because bone must be weakened before it can be strengthened, runners who increase their mileage too quickly often develop small bone

fissures that cause increasing amounts of pain. Once these microfissures surpass a certain degree of concentration and severity, a stress fracture results. The pain of a stress fracture is usually so severe that running becomes unthinkable.

Training through It

It is usually easy to avoid bone strains by reducing your running as soon as you start to experience shin pain. Wait for the pain to subside and then cautiously resume your mileage ramp-up. Don't be surprised if you have to repeat this process a second time before your bones have become strong enough to handle all the running you care to do.

In the meantime, cross-train in alternative cardiovascular activities that you can do pain-free. One option is "running" very slowly on a treadmill set to maximum incline (a 15 percent grade on a typical machine). This variation has a couple of key advantages. First, it reduces impact to a level that does not exacerbate or interfere with the healing of mild bone strains. Nevertheless, because it is a low-impact, weight-bearing activity, it keeps the bones stronger than other running alternatives, such as bicycling, that are non-weight-bearing. If you spend a lot of time cross-training exclusively in non-weight-bearing activities, you will face a high risk of suffering another bone strain when you return to running because bone adaptations to running begin to reverse themselves when weight-bearing exercise ceases. Another advantage of slow treadmill running on a very steep incline is that it is more similar to running than cycling and other alternatives are, so there is more of a fitness crossover back to normal running.

Tibial bone strains and stress fractures are more likely to occur in women with low bone mineral density and in those with naturally thin bones. Running itself is a great way to build bone density, but only if you avoid doing too much too soon and if you support your running with a proper diet. Consuming adequate total calories, avoiding carbonated soft drinks, eating plenty of vegetables, and taking calcium supplements will help strengthen your bones. There's nothing you can do about naturally thin bones, however.

As you might expect, research has shown that runners whose stride mechanics expose their legs to greater impact forces are more likely to develop tibial stress fractures. You may be able to reduce your risk of bone strains and stress fractures by altering your stride to reduce impact severity. In a small study, gait retraining expert Irene Davis of the University of Delaware was able to train previous sufferers of stress fractures to significantly reduce their impact using force plates and biofeedback. She believes that runners can achieve a similar effect on their own by listening to the sound of their footstrikes and modifying their strides to make them quieter. This is done by activating the muscles earlier and to a greater degree, which reduces the load on the bone. If you're a heel-striker, modifying your stride so that you land on the midfoot should also reduce impact forces and your injury risk.

Shoe characteristics also affect impact forces, but as we explained earlier, they do so in somewhat unpredictable ways that differ from runner to runner. Again, we can only suggest that you consider your shoes a possible contributor to any bone strain or stress fracture you suffer and see whether you can find a more comfortable pair of running shoes to replace them.

Finally, there is some evidence that runners who have experienced stress fractures are more likely to exhibit muscle imbalances in their lower legs. These muscles help absorb impact forces and must be strong and flexible to do their job effectively. The eccentric heel dip, described on page 59, will strengthen your calf muscle–Achilles tendon complex. The ankle mobilization exercise described in the previous section on plantar fasciitis will enhance the flexibility of this complex. To strengthen the ankle dorsiflexors on the front of your shins and improve sensory feedback control of your lower-leg muscles, try balancing on a balance board or disk such as the Reebok Core Board. These tools are available at many sporting goods stores.

ACHILLES TENDINOSIS

Achilles tendinosis used to be called "Achilles tendinitis," back when medical scientists believed that it was fundamentally an inflammatory condition. But its name changed when it was discovered that the real problem is tissue degeneration resulting from repeated tendon strain.

Description and Causes

During running, the Achilles tendon may be exposed to forces equaling 8 to 10 times the runner's body weight. The resulting strain may cause microtrauma that does not always have a chance to fully heal between training sessions. The injured tendon heals by "bandaging" the damaged area with a type of collagen that is much stiffer than the dominant type of collagen in the tendon, making the tendon less elastic and even more prone to damage during continued running.

Interestingly, the stiffer type of collagen gradually replaces the more elastic type as one ages, which probably explains why older runners are more susceptible to Achilles tendinosis. It has also been proposed that the injury occurs more commonly in faster runners and in runners currently increasing their volume of high-intensity running, which makes sense, because stresses on the Achilles tendon increase dramatically with increased speed. And finally, if you have experienced any Achilles tendinopathy, you might have your parents to thank. Some recent research has demonstrated a genetic basis for this condition, and although having a parent or relative who has experienced tendinosis will not guarantee that you get it, it is reason to be more wary of any niggling sensations you feel in that area.

Runners usually first notice pain at the beginning or end of runs. If training continues, pain spreads during the run and becomes increasingly intense. Fast running and uphill running are especially painful. You may also feel pain when you climb stairs, stand on your toes, and so forth.

Treatment and Rehabilitation

When these symptoms emerge, immediately reduce your running to a pain-free amount, slow down and avoid hills, as necessary. Icing will not help, because inflammation is not the problem, and NSAIDs slow the healing process, so avoid them.

The most effective treatment for Achilles tendinosis is eccentric calf muscle strengthening. Swedish orthopedist Hakan Alfredson purportedly attempted to rupture his Achilles tendon intentionally by doing eccentric calf exercises with heavy loads, only to find that these exercises resolved his symptoms!

Begin your eccentric calf muscle strengthening program only when you can do unweighted eccentric heel dips with minimal pain. Introduce weight as soon as you are strong enough and you can do so without additional pain, and continue increasing the load as you become stronger.

There is some experimental evidence and a good deal of clinical evidence that Achilles tendinosis responds well to a special type of massage known as transverse friction massage. In this technique, the tissues of the Achilles tendon and calf muscles are rubbed against the grain of their fibers under deep pressure.

PART 2

The Cardioresp

iratory System

In Part 1 we took a detailed look at the organization of the body from a single cell all the way up to the whole organism, and what we learned was that it is the organ systems of the body working together that allow us to survive. Then we examined the musculoskeletal system, and one of the themes of that entire section was human movement and how the muscles must contract to allow us to run. But the muscles need energy to perform their work, and you must always remember that although we organize the body into pieces, these individual pieces always function in unison and are mutually exclusive—that is, if one of them is compromised, the body will cope for a period of time but eventually will not survive. So the muscles need energy to do their job. In Chapter 8, you will learn that we obtain the required energy from both carbohydrates and fats, but for now we are going to examine exactly what the cardiovascular and cardiorespiratory systems do so that your muscles enable you to make the movements that allow you to run.

The Lungs

With global warming and deforestation hot topics in our world today, we often hear how the Amazon rain forest, with its millions of trees, is "the lungs of the planet." Where does this analogy come from? The ideas of respiration and ventilation are the keys to understanding how our cardiorespiratory system works. The first term, *respiration,* refers to the uptake of oxygen (O_2) and the production of carbon dioxide (CO_2). In the plant world, respiration means the uptake of CO_2 and the production of O_2, but the central theme is the same in that one is going in, and the cells are using it, and the other one is coming out as a by-product.

It is probably safe to assume that you realize the importance of O_2 to your body. All your cells need it, especially muscle during running, but it is something that we do not produce in the body and therefore must extract from the air. *Ventilation* is how we accomplish this. Ventilation is the process of moving air in and out of our lungs by breathing so that we can take oxygen from the air and get it into our blood. Then the cardiovascular system takes over and delivers the O_2 to the body's tissues and organs through circulation.

In the cardiorespiratory system, the lungs and the heart (separate organs) work together. As we ventilate and move air over the lungs' large surface area (1,100 square feet in total, or about the size of a small apartment), we extract O_2 from that air, and it moves into the blood. The nuts and bolts of it are quite complex, and fortunately there is no need to delve into them here. The best thing is that you do not need to think about breathing. It is driven by changes in O_2 and especially CO_2 in the blood, and your body does the rest to ensure that everything remains within the desired range.

However, the battle is only half won at this point, as that is only the "respiratory" part of the system. The "cardio" aspect entails the heart and how it takes blood returning from the body and sends it to the lungs, where we dump the CO_2 and swap it with O_2. Then the lungs send the oxygen-rich blood back to the heart to be carried to the rest of the body's tissues.

The Cardiovascular System

In the cardiovascular system, the heart also teams up with all the blood vessels (the "vascular" element), which serve as the plumbing of the body and form a network of "pipes" throughout the tissues. For the runner, the heart's ability to pump blood to the body and nourish itself is crucial. In fact, as you become more trained, your heart adapts and pumps more blood with each stroke, and therefore more blood per minute. Also, the system is a closed loop with a pump maintaining pressure. This is also crucial: Too much pressure and the heart works too hard; too little pressure and insufficient blood (and O_2)is delivered to the tissues. A couple of things can affect the pressure in profound ways. The first is the volume of the blood; specifically, if we lower the volume, the pressure goes down. Thankfully this is seldom a problem, and a drop in blood volume large enough to affect pressure occurs only in traumatic situations that result in profound blood loss. The other is related to the diameter of the blood vessels. As we make the diameter larger, the pressure drops, and as we make it smaller, the pressure rises. One of the remarkable aspects of our cardiovascular system is that it can control the diameter of these blood vessels, and in doing so, it can adjust the pressure so that it can always deliver enough blood and O_2 to the tissues.

Managing Supply and Demand

The muscular aspect of running is quite complex, as your brain activates and relaxes different muscles in just the right order to produce a nice stride. But equally remarkable is how your body meets the increased energy demand of the muscles by making changes in how you breathe (both faster and deeper) and how you deliver the O_2 and take away the CO_2 (increasing your heart rate and opening up more blood vessels). We are now going to take a look at some different aspects of the cardiorespiratory system and the cardiovascular system, and how these two systems play a role in your running.

Chapter 5

More Mileage per Milliliter

In the 1997 film *Gattaca*, Vincent Freeman, the character played by Ethan Hawke, finds himself with a dilemma: He is one of the unlucky ones who don't possess the perfect DNA that is required to enable them to travel in space. Vincent has a congenital heart condition that rules him out in a society that analyzes every person's DNA to determine their life expectancy and their likelihood of disease. So Vincent has to assume the identity of a genetically perfect but crippled man, Jerome, to achieve prominence and fulfill his dream of space travel.

Runners often find themselves in a similar dilemma, except that instead of having their future prospects limited by their DNA, they're often told that their VO_2 max—the maximum volume of oxygen that your muscles can use when you are running at the fastest speed you can sustain for a period of time—is too low to allow them to be successful runners. Runners are taught that their VO_2 max determines their standing in the running universe. Just as your platinum credit card signifies your financial and social standing, your VO_2 max is the numerical expression of your *Gattaca*-like chances of successful running.

VO_2 max has long been regarded as the definitive predictor of running ability. It's certainly one of the best and most widely used measures of cardiorespiratory capacity and is often assumed to be a limiting factor in exercise performance, an assumption we'll discuss in greater detail in Chapter 11, in the fatigue section.

The highest VO_2 max values are typically measured in runners and cross-country skiers, because these sports involve the use of arm, trunk, and leg muscles. More active muscle involvement means more oxygen use, hence a higher VO_2. Generally, elite runners have VO_2 max values between 65 milliliters per kilogram per minute (ml/kg/min) and 85 ml/kg/min. This wide range is a clue that VO_2 max is not necessarily all it's cracked up to be, because if it were so crucial, then one would expect all the elite to be clustered around the higher end of this range. Competition would also be irrelevant—champions could be crowned in the laboratory, and this is clearly not the case.

One reason for the exaggerated importance of the relationship between VO_2 max and performance is that VO_2 max is so easy to measure and quantify. Some of the other recognized factors in running success, such as muscle-tendon elasticity, the ability to use fat as fuel, and the capacity to generate ATP at rapid rates, are a lot more difficult to measure and often impossible to quantify or compare from one runner to the next. The attraction of finding a single value that determines your running ability is too great to resist, so the notion that VO_2 max is the physiological stand-in for running potential has become dogma among runners and some exercise physiologists, despite the abundant evidence that performance is far more complex than what a single number might suggest.

Effect of training: The Physiology of VO_2 Max

Inasmuch as we do accept the importance of VO_2 max, the obvious question we must ask is whether VO_2 max can be substantially improved by training, or whether we are consigned to a life of mediocrity as a result of having poorly chosen our parents. The answer is fairly complex and only mildly encouraging. Jim Ryun, one of America's most famous milers, was reported to have a VO_2 max of 82 ml/kg/min at his peak and a value of "only" 65 ml/kg/min after a year without training. This suggests that he could increase his VO_2 max by 26 percent. This data is somewhat anecdotal and doesn't account for many years of cumulative training and their possible effect on that starting value of 65 ml/kg/min, which might not represent a true baseline measurement.

For a more systematic view of the effects of training on VO_2 max—one that is more relevant to all of us sub–Jim Ryun–caliber runners—we need to look elsewhere. Clues come from the famous HERITAGE Family Study, in which five universities in the United States collaborated to perform research on physiological adaptations to exercise training. The study looked at 481 sedentary individuals from 98 two-generation families (thus enabling them to assess how genetics influenced the adaptations) and their responses to a 20-week exercise-training program.

Researchers found that there was enormous heterogeneity in the response of VO$_2$ max to training. In other words, the response of the body to training varies hugely from one individual to the next. For example, 20 weeks of training increased VO$_2$ max by an average of 400 ml/min, or about 16 percent. However, some individuals were able to increase their VO$_2$ max by more than 1,000 ml/min (40 percent), while others achieved no change at all. Most intriguingly, the "responders" to training, those who did achieve large increases in VO$_2$ max, tended to be from the same family but were not necessarily the individuals who had high VO$_2$ max values to begin with. In other words, the capacity to adapt to training is genetically determined but is not influenced in the same way as the genetically determined baseline. Therefore, not only do the genes influence the starting level for VO$_2$ max, but they also independently affect how responsive VO$_2$ max is to endurance training.

To further understand the effects of training on VO$_2$ max, we must first consider which physiological factors influence VO$_2$ max and then how the VO$_2$ max value is measured. For such a ubiquitous and important measurement, the physiology underlying the concept of VO$_2$ max is still hotly debated. To oversimplify the argument, the maximal capacity of the body to use oxygen is thought to be determined first by the ability of the heart to pump

oxygen-rich blood to the muscles and second by the ability of the muscles to extract that oxygen from the blood for use. Therefore, VO$_2$ max is usually said to be limited by the capacity of the cardiovascular system, though there is much debate as to whether it is the heart, the lungs, or the muscles that have the greatest influence.

Large, strong lungs that are capable of delivering oxygen to the blood and a large, strong heart that can pump blood to the muscles during peak exercise combine in elite athletes to satisfy the first requirement for a high VO$_2$ max. Elite athletes are able to increase the total volume of blood pumped per minute (called the cardiac output) from about 5 liters at rest to close to 40 liters at maximum effort, thanks to enormous increases in stroke volume (the amount of blood pumped per contraction) and heart rate. Combined with large, efficient lungs and blood that is rich in hemoglobin to carry oxygen, cardiac output capacity ensures the ability to deliver oxygen very effectively to the exercising muscles. Part of the body's response to training is to increase all three of these factors: Your heart and lungs become bigger and stronger, and the capacity of your blood to carry oxygen increases.

When oxygen reaches the muscle, it is taken out of the blood and used in chemical reactions to produce energy in the form of ATP. This extraction represents the other proposed site of limitation in oxygen use, with factors such as enzyme activity failure and molecular-level impaired muscle function defining that limit. These factors could combine to prevent the muscle from using all of the available oxygen.

A more recent, contrary argument states that VO_2 max is in fact not limited by the cardiorespiratory system at all. Instead, the argument proposes that VO_2 max is a nonlimiting symptom of regulatory control by another independent system: the brain, which regulates exercise intensity. Because exercise intensity determines how much muscle is active, the use of oxygen is a reflection of the regulation of muscle activity, rather than the factor that determines it. This paradigm shift requires that VO_2 max be viewed not as the predictor of performance but rather as a measurable indicator of how exercise is regulated.

To further appreciate this argument, you need to understand how VO_2 max is actually measured in the laboratory. Usually, the athlete being tested will perform a treadmill running trial (or another aerobic activity, such as stationary cycling) to exhaustion in a laboratory. The athlete begins at a slow, jogging pace, and the speed is increased every minute or two until the athlete can no longer keep up with the treadmill belt and must choose to stop (or be propelled off the back of the treadmill!).

In this protocol, what is happening physiologically is that the athlete is being forced to activate more and more muscle to meet the demand for increasing running speed. The slow speeds at the start require low levels of muscle activation, whereas at the end (with speeds often as high as 14 to 15 mph for elite runners), much more muscle must be activated. A rise in exercise intensity is achieved by increasing the total number of active muscle fibers. The ever-increasing activation of muscle is responsible for driving the increasing use of oxygen. Ultimately, then, rather than the *cause* of the high running speed, the maximal oxygen consumption, or VO_2 max, is a function of both running speed and the muscle activation required to achieve that speed. In other words, fast runners don't run fast because they are able to consume a lot of oxygen; rather, they consume a lot of oxygen because they are able to run fast. Was Jim Ryun able to run faster when his VO_2 max was 82 ml/kg/min than when it was 65 ml/kg/min? Undoubtedly, yes. But was the higher VO_2 max the cause of this ability? No, it was merely the measure of something else—his training status at that moment, which allowed him to achieve faster running speeds, greater muscle activation, and, hence, a higher VO_2 max value during the test.

There are, of course, individual characteristics that modulate this relationship, which is why two people running at the same speed seldom use equal volumes of oxygen.

Nevertheless, if we want to consider how training might affect VO_2 max, then this change in paradigm becomes crucial. Instead of training to improve our capacity to consume oxygen so we can run faster, we now want to train to activate more muscle tissue so we can run faster. The capacity to activate a lot of muscle tissue when running is determined not only by training but by genetic inheritance as well.

Introducing Running Economy

All is not lost, however, for those not blessed with the highest VO_2 max in their running club, because there are a number of other factors that are acknowledged as crucial determinants of running ability. Perhaps the most provocative and least understood is running economy. Running economy refers to how efficiently your body uses oxygen when you are running at submaximal speeds.

A quick peek into the sport of cycling helps us appreciate just how important economy is. It has been found that the most successful cyclists (in terms of achievement) do not necessarily have the highest VO_2 max values. Instead, they are highly efficient and possess a remarkable ability to use minimal oxygen during cycling at all speeds. Efficiency and economy differ subtly, and the difference is not worth picking apart here. The key point is

that some athletes—runners as well as cyclists—are able to do more work with a given volume of oxygen than others; they have greater economy.

The implication of economy for VO_2 max is somewhat ironic, because a more economical runner who uses less oxygen is destined to have a lower VO_2 max than an inefficient cyclist, no matter what the speed. Therefore a high VO_2 max might actually predict *poor* performance in endurance events, because it suggests that the athlete is less efficient. Of course, this is not entirely true, and what you really want is either to have both a very high VO_2 max and great efficiency or to possess the hybrid capacity to produce a lot of energy very efficiently.

Economy is no more the end-all of running performance than VO_2 max is, but it is equally important—and as little understood as it is important. So let's take a much closer look at the phenomenon of running economy.

Running Economy 101

Running economy is increasingly being recognized as crucial to running success, though our understanding of it is still limited and shrouded in confusion and ambiguity. Considering how important running economy seems to be, it has surprisingly been somewhat ignored in the literature.

In 2007, a high-powered gathering of exercise physiologists and scientists convened in

Chicago for a conference on Marathon Medicine and Physiology, where the topic of running economy was tackled once again. At that conference, Carl Foster, one of the authors of a fascinating research study that examined the running economy of Zersenay Tadese (see page 84), discussed the role of running economy in performance. He suggested that science has "ignored running economy" to date, despite being aware of it for 30 years, and, as a result, relatively little is known about the topic.

One thing we do know is that by becoming a more economical runner, you'll become a better one. But what does running economy measure? And how does it affect performance? And, most important of all, how do you improve it? These are the relevant questions that need to be tackled to help you get "more mileage per milliliter" of oxygen.

A Closer Look

When we talk about running economy, we are referring to how much oxygen the body uses at a given running speed. Remember that oxygen is used by the muscles to produce energy, so measuring oxygen use is a proxy for measuring energy use. Running economy is probably analogous to cruising efficiency in a car, since it concerns how much fuel is being used at a given submaximal speed rather than at maximal speed or acceleration.

This submaximal context is important, because when you think about it, the idea that endurance running performance is limited by maximal oxygen doesn't quite ring true for any running event that doesn't get you above that oxygen ceiling. That is, you might have an incredibly high VO_2 max when you're running at top speeds, but how is this relevant when you run a marathon? Or even a 10-K race? In fact, any run longer than about 5 kilometers is run below the VO_2 max running speed, so the "limit" is not reached.

Chapter 11 presents a detailed discussion of the origins of fatigue, but it's worth mentioning at this stage that a prevalent theory of exercise fatigue says that you slow down because the muscles' demand for oxygen exceeds the available supply. The result is that your muscles become *anaerobic*—starved of oxygen—and are eventually unable to contract as effectively. This theory is challenged in detail later, but for now, let's assume it to be true. If this is the case, why then would a marathon runner even care about VO_2 max, when he's running at only 80 percent of his maximum? Even if it existed, that anaerobic limit simply would not be relevant to most running events. So while a high VO_2 max is a good thing, a high running economy is an even better thing in race distances exceeding 5 kilometers.

Running Economy Explained and Applied

Let's briefly turn our attention to an illustration of running economy, together with some examples from the elite, which reinforce the concept that it's how little oxygen you use, not how much, that is most important to your running performance.

Consider the hypothetical (and somewhat contrived, for simplicity's sake) example of Alex and Dave, shown below.

Alex and Dave (who weigh the same, by the way) are tested in an exercise physiology lab, where the amount of oxygen they use while running at a range of speeds from 5 minutes per kilometer (min/km) to 3 min/

km is measured. Starting with the highest speed, we discover that when Alex and Dave are running as fast as possible, they use the same volume of oxygen: 66 ml/kg/min.

If you move left along the graphs and look at the slower running speeds, you'll see that Alex and Dave are no longer similar: Alex uses less oxygen than Dave at all of these slower speeds. This means that Alex has a better running economy. And because Alex is using less oxygen and energy at a given speed, he has the potential to run

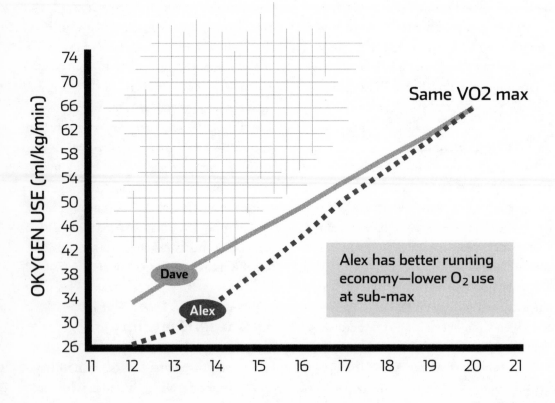

OXYGEN USE (ml/kg/min)

Same VO2 max

Dave

Alex

Alex has better running economy—lower O$_2$ use at sub-max

slightly faster than Dave before he reaches the limit where he's using as much oxygen and energy as he can without fatigue before his running task is completed. Using the analogy of fuel economy in cars, the more economical the car, the faster you can go while still burning the same total fuel volume. In a race between Alex and Dave, the smart money will bet on Alex because he can run that little bit faster before energy use or oxygen delivery begins to become important as a performance limiter.

We see this phenomenon all the time outside the laboratory and the realm of hypothetical runners. In elite athletes, VO_2 max very rarely predicts who will win races. For example, Kenyan runners, who dominate distance running, have VO_2 max values that are often lower than those of the Europeans they run against. In fact, if you used the VO_2 max values of the top 50 runners in the world as your sole criteria for ranking the athletes for performance ability, you'd have about the same degree of accuracy as if you stuck a list of names on the wall and ranked them by throwing darts into it. In this narrow group, VO_2 max tends to have little impact on performance. Sometimes the best performance comes from the athlete with the lowest VO_2 max, precisely because he or she is the most economical.

By contrast, differences in running economy do explain some variations in performance ability, even among elite runners. The graph on page 86, based on numerous studies on running economy, depicts the running economy of American, European, and East African runners at a range of running speeds. Note that the y-axis shows economy as oxygen used *per kilometer*, which is a somewhat different unit of measurement from that used to express VO_2 max, expressed as *volume per minute*. Here, researchers are looking at the total volume of oxygen used by the runner to complete 1 kilometer. What they've found is that an East African typically uses 180 ml/kg to run 1 kilometer at a speed of 20 kilometers per hour. This is relatively easy to translate into a volume per minute, because you know that at this speed, 1 kilometer takes three minutes; the VO_2 is thus 60 ml/kg/min.

This graph shows quite clearly that the East African runners have an economy advantage over the European and American runners, which is an exciting finding for those wishing to understand why almost every distance world record in athletics is held by an East African. Exactly what explains this advantage is more difficult to determine. It is probably a combination of molecular, biomechanical, anatomical, and physiological factors. Some of these are discussed later, together with training ideas to improve running economy, but it certainly does appear that, as with cycling, the best runners are those who are able to get more mileage per milliliter of oxygen.

We don't want to overstate our case. While it may be greater economy that separates the East African runners from other world-class runners, you'd be very hard pressed to find any world-class runner with a VO_2 max lower than about 70 ml/kg/min. And although a high VO_2 max is a consequence rather than a cause of the ability to run fast, there is no doubt that the ability to run fast results in part from a strong cardiovascular system. In the past, scientists have oversimplified exercise physiology by considering a strong cardiovascular system the

be-all and end-all of endurance performance. We don't want to commit the mirror image of this mistake by arguing that economy is the true be-all and end-all. A strong cardiorespiratory system and a high level of efficiency are equally important to running performance, as are other factors discussed elsewhere in this book. Exercise physiology is far too complex to be boiled down to a single secret to success.

Without a doubt, though, running economy is one of the many secrets. The best runners tend to be the most economical; certain physiological characteristics predispose runners to be more economical; and certain types

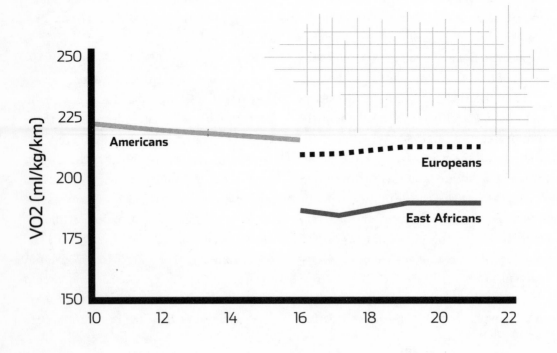

of training improve running economy more than others.

The Components of Running Economy

What are the components that contribute to creating an economical runner? We've recognized that certain runners, despite having "inferior" VO_2 max values, are still competitive, or even dominant, because they are able to use oxygen more effectively than others. The question is why. Are some people born economical, or do a few months of targeted training bring you in line with the most economical runners in the world?

The truth is that we don't really know. Our knowledge of the underpinnings of running economy is still a long way from where it should be. Our good friend Amby Burfoot, *Runner's World* magazine editor at large, is fond of reminding us that science is actually a long way from understanding running physiology in general, and he's quite right. In the words of Sir Roger Bannister, the first man to crack the four-minute mile, who then went on to become a respected neurologist, "The human body is centuries in advance of the physiologist, and can perform an integration of heart, lungs, and muscles which is too complex for the scientist to analyze."

Running economy is one such "integration." With that idea in mind, let's unpack the parts and see whether we might be able to "build" ourselves an economical runner.

BIOMECHANICAL FACTORS INFLUENCING RUNNING ECONOMY

According to an excellent 2004 review article by M. Saunders of Penn State, the following biomechanical factors are important for running economy:

→ **Height:** Slightly smaller-than-average height is advantageous for men, while slightly taller is better for women. We must confess that we don't have an explanation for the difference, and we suspect that if the research net is cast a little more widely to include more data, this difference might disappear.

→ **Somatotype:** Runners with an ectomorphic physique demonstrate the best running economy. An ectomorph is generally long-limbed and thin, with shoulders that are about the same width as the hips. Think Paul Tergat, or just about any other Kenyan long-distance runner.

→ **Body fat:** A low percentage is ideal, because body fat represents additional weight that must be carried, increasing the oxygen cost of running.

→ **Leg morphology:** Most of the runner's weight should be distributed closer to the hips. In other words, if you have mass, it's best if it's carried in the quads and not the calves, since weight in the calves exerts an effect on the torque needed to accelerate and decelerate the limbs, requiring increased oxygen use. A research study from 2007 found that Zersenay Tadese, Eritrea's cross-country world champion, had the best running economy ever measured, at only 150 ml/kg/km. It was speculated that this economical number could be accounted for in part by the very small size of his calves compared with those of the European runners with whom he was compared.

→ **Pelvis:** A narrow pelvis, as is the case in ectomorphs, is an advantage.

→ **Feet:** Smaller-than-average feet contribute to economy.

→ **Shoes:** Lightweight but well-cushioned shoes improve running economy, possibly because cushioning reduces the work required by the muscles to absorb and cushion the landing.

→ **Stride length:** Freely chosen. This finding is interesting, because there is evidence from research that if you chop, or shorten, your stride to try to increase the cadence, your running economy worsens. We cover this topic in Chapter 12, but there is a recent trend for runners to force increased cadence, aiming for 90 strides per minute. This often requires a chopping of the stride, which is undesirable according to the economy research.

Having said that, overstriding is just as bad, if not worse, for your running economy, because a great deal of energy is lost to braking when you land with your foot well in front of your center of mass. Stride length, perhaps more than anything else, emphasizes that practice makes perfect and that running is a skill that must be practiced and learned. Comfortable, efficient strides happen naturally, yes, but must be learned and very subtly modified by informed feedback, rather than through wholesale changes in a one-size-fits-all approach.

→ **Kinematics:** Minimal vertical oscillation of the center of mass is desirable. What does this mean? Well, it means don't waste energy going up and down if you don't need to. The less energy you expend on vertical braking forces, the better. The most economical runners scoot forward with minimal vertical oscillation by effectively "rolling" their legs along beneath their bodies. There is nothing new about this; we've known for a long time that a relatively flat trajectory is more economical.

Minimizing arm movement also enhances running economy. Some movement is better than none, because the arms play an important role in providing rotational stability, but the movement must not be excessive. Having said this, we recognize there are some absolutely bizarre arm carries among the elite runners, which we'd have thought would be corrected in training, so it's clear that there's more than one effective way to use the arms when running.

A more acute knee angle during the swing phase of the stride is another economy booster. In other words, when your trailing leg is coming through (e.g., your right foot is planted on the ground and your left leg is swinging through), then it's better to have that knee fully bent rather than slightly bent or straight. The reasons for this are grounded in physics and relate to rotational torque and the force that is required from the quadriceps muscles to bring the leg through. But the practical point is that the hamstrings come into play with regard to running economy, because they contribute to the flexing of the knees. One practical point here is that when you run slowly, it's almost impossible to bend the knees more than a few degrees—you'd be working so hard to bend your knees, you'd increase your energy cost instead of reducing it. So the desirability of a folded swing leg is largely influenced by running speed.

The take-home point from the above list is that if you are a skinny man, weighing next to nothing, with hips as wide as your shoulders, short arms, and no body fat, and you wear a well-cushioned pair of size 5 shoes, you might have good running economy.

Seriously, though, the most important thing that jumps out from the above list is that there are some factors that one is born with (height, pelvis width, foot size, distribution of weight on the legs) and others that are improved with training and preparation, such as the kinematics of vertical oscillation and arm carry. The list also does not account for metabolic factors, such as the use of oxygen at the cellular level, which is undoubtedly improved with training. The bottom line is that great runners are born and then trained. Since every runner can train, there is probably a great deal that you can do to improve your running economy, which would then translate into improved performance. We need to consider those factors that we can control and then decide how best to incorporate focused training into our programs to make a difference in our running.

TRAINING AND RUNNING ECONOMY

For all the research on running economy and its obvious importance to running performance, there is still confusion about which type of training has the biggest impact on economy, and the issue has been surprisingly underresearched. We remind you that running economy was called the "forgotten" variable by one prominent expert (Carl Foster). Also, the initial level of fitness and ability of the runner plays a huge role, as we're sure you can appreciate—a good runner needs very different training compared with a novice. So it can be somewhat tricky to tease out the valuable information.

However, considering that running economy is a measure of how efficiently you use oxygen, it stands to reason that in order to improve it, you must eliminate all wasteful movements and muscle contractions that consume oxygen without helping you move forward. Evidence suggests that the most effective training to improve running economy is simply to run—the more the better, as long as you stay within your personal limits. The speed doesn't matter, and in one sense slower running is better, because you can spend more time running slowly than you can running fast. Just as you would train so your golf swing or a dance move became more efficient and controlled through repetitive movement, so, too, you need to "teach" your brain and muscles how to be most efficient.

This point may represent a bit of a shift in thinking, because we don't often think of running as a technical skill that is learned and improved like golf. And perhaps it's better left that way—the last thing you want to do on your easy five-mile loop is overanalyze your technique. Luckily for us, the body is able to learn without our consciously worrying about it; the brain and the muscles (called the neuromuscular system) are able to adapt naturally and improve the efficiency of movement in the course of normal training.

As suggested above, however, the type of training that is most beneficial to running economy depends on your individual experience and fitness level. If you are relatively new to running, then you benefit the most from endurance training: longer duration, slower running. However, if you're relatively experienced and already do a fair amount of longer running, then the addition of some speed and strength work will make an impact.

One of the things that change with regular running is that your body "learns" to be more economical by reducing the distance you move up and down during the stride. Recall from the list provided earlier that vertical oscillation is a key predictor of running economy. Well, it so happens that training reduces vertical oscillation, and thus improves running economy. In addition, there are all kinds of metabolic and cardiovascular changes that contribute to improved running economy, including production of more mitochondria in the muscles, which helps you use oxygen and produce energy more effectively.

The essential message, then, is to use longer, slower distance running to ramp up your running economy—practice makes perfect. But after that, use longer, slower work for maintenance and consider the addition of some speedwork and strength training to improve your performance and economy even more.

THE IMPORTANCE OF SPEEDWORK

Studies have looked at middle-distance (800 meters to 1500 meters) runners and found that they are more economical than marathon runners at faster speeds, simply because they are accustomed to those speeds. Running economy improves most at the specific paces that are trained most—an observation that points to the importance of neuromuscular coordination for running economy. This is why, with your 50-minute, 10-kilometer best time, you feel relatively comfortable at 5 min/km. As soon as you enter the 4 min/km range, however, you may feel that you are floundering and losing control of your own movements. It's simply that your neuromuscular system is unused to that speed of movement, and you lack the coordination required to run efficiently at the faster speed.

Given this observation, it is logical to speculate that if you can become more economical at faster speeds, your economy will improve at slower speeds. And research suggests that this is true, to a degree. If you do regular speedwork, you will become more economical across the whole range of running paces. The interesting thing is that the effect is lost if you do too much faster-paced running. In fact, excessive speedwork may even make you less economical at slower speeds. So the best recipe for improved running economy is a balanced program that includes runs at a variety of paces and one or two speed sessions per week.

STRENGTH AND PLYOMETRICS

Finally, one of the most interesting and undervalued forms of training for runners, proven to enhance economy, is strength work. This includes a special type of strength training known as plyometrics, which involves jumping drills and is explained in more detail on page 93.

Strength training and plyometrics have both been shown to improve running performance and economy. They probably do so by taking advantage of something known as the stretch-shortening cycle (SSC). The stretch-shortening cycle refers to the transition between two different types of muscle contractions that occur during running and how elastic energy is used to assist with force production.

As your foot lands on the ground, various muscles lengthen in what is called an *eccentric* muscle contraction. This stretching of the muscles captures energy from the force of impact, much as a stretched rubber band captures the energy you put into stretching it. As soon as you push off, these same muscles shorten in what is called a *concentric* muscle contraction. The concentric contraction is more powerful and more efficient if it closely follows the eccentric contraction, because it is able to use more of that captured energy, which quickly dissipates if the pause between stretching and shortening is too long. A muscle with a quick stretch-shortening cycle therefore uses less oxygen and energy to produce the same level of force. This is why if you want to jump up as high as possible (for example, to slam-dunk a basketball), you first drop down into a squat and then bounce back up, taking advantage of the stretch-shortening cycle to improve the performance of your jump.

During running, the stretch-shortening cycle is critical to performance and running economy. The muscle contracts in the milliseconds before the foot hits the ground. This muscle contraction is known as *preactivation*, and it serves the vital purpose of increasing the stiffness of the muscle-tendon unit. A stiff muscle-tendon unit is able to store and return energy far more effectively than would be the case in the absence of muscle activation. (Think of the elastic recoil of a stiff golf ball compared with a mushy squash ball, for example.) The result of preactivation is that the energy stored in the eccentric landing phase is used in the concentric push-off, reducing the contact time with the ground and, in theory, improving running economy and performance.

Researchers in Finland have extensively examined how plyometric training affects running economy and performance. First, they established that during the course of a five-kilometer time trial, the degree of muscle preactivation gradually declined, and ground contact time went up. As a result, the runners' speed decreased. They then looked at how various types of training affected five-kilometer performance, finding that only four weeks of plyometric training improved performance significantly. The mechanism for this improvement is probably neuromuscular, because they found that the plyometrically trained athletes had a greater degree of preactivation than untrained athletes; this translated into an 8 percent reduction in ground contact time and an 8 percent decrease in oxygen use during the time trial. It appears that the plyometric training improved running performance and economy by stimulating these neuromuscular adaptations.

The fact that speed and power training improve running economy most, suggests that perhaps the answers to improved performance lie not in the heart and lungs but in the muscles and tendons. It also suggests the possibility that the biggest differences between us and the world's best runners lie in the muscles and tendons rather than in the heart and lungs.

You can spot those runners who have an efficient neuromuscular system; they seem to be bouncing along, touching the ground very lightly, with minimal contact time, as though they are running on eggshells. We have little doubt that this spring effect is the biggest factor contributing to the dominance of East Africans in running. They have superior "springs," and their energy cost of running is much lower as a result.

Strength training, particularly plyometric training, has been found to improve running economy in a short space of time, probably by exaggerating and improving the energy return from muscle and tendon. There is more than one way to practice plyometric training. Sometimes hill running is sufficient; other times, you can get creative and come up with all sorts of drills, using hurdles, ropes, and your imagination. Having said all this, we must warn you against overdoing plyometrics as the "secret weapon" in your training. The risk of injury is relatively high, so these drills should neither be attempted by novice runners nor done too often. Do them perhaps once a week at first and never more than twice a week.

FLEXIBILITY

Another attribute relevant to running economy is flexibility, but its influence is very different from that of a fast stretch-shortening cycle. There was a time when runners were continuously drilled to do as much stretching as possible. Failure to do so, we were told, would predispose us to injury. Well, injuries aside, there is evidence that being too flexible negatively affects running economy and possibly performance.

There is much confusion about this matter, however. One study, for example, found that improving the flexibility of the hip flexors and extensors resulted in better running economy. The explanation for this was that if your hips are flexible enough, provided hip flexibility is balanced between left and right, front and back, then you need to do less work to balance and stabilize your body during running. This explanation lacks plausibility for reasons we will share momentarily.

Other research has found that being less flexible is better for running economy. In fact, a preponderance of studies show that "tighter" runners are more economical than "looser" runners. For example, in novice runners all the way to elite runners, it's been found that as flexibility in the trunk (hips and core muscles) and the legs increases, running economy decreases. Therefore, if you want to be economical, err on the side of being inflexible.

The explanation behind these findings is far more believable, according to theoretical insights. We've discussed how the stiffness and ability of the muscle to store and then release energy helps with running and reduces oxygen cost. Flexibility works against this characteristic. If you are very flexible in the legs (especially the calves and ankles), then you need to do far more to stabilize your joints and store energy, and so it pays to be stiffer and less flexible. Similarly, the less flexible you are in the trunk muscles, the more stable the pelvis is and the less muscle work is required to limit unwanted motion as you run—you're a more "compact unit," so to speak. To sum it up: Less flexibility means less work is required for stability, and elastic energy return from stiffer muscles and joints increases. This only makes sense. Training tends to reduce the flexibility of some joints. Why would running stimulate this adaptation if it reduced performance, when every other adaptation that it stimulates— from growth of the heart muscle to increased sweating capacity—is known to enhance performance?

This doesn't mean that flexibility is not important. You certainly must have a normal range of motion in your joints to run efficiently. But any extra range of motion is wasteful. Balance in your range of motion matters most. Your right hip needs to extend as efficiently as your left hip does, and both hips need to flex as well as they extend. It's best therefore to avoid random, indiscriminate stretching, because for all you know, you're messing up your natural balance, increasing injury risk, and becoming less economical. Do just enough stretching to stay balanced, and leave it there. Everything in moderation!

Conclusion

Few aspects of running physiology are at once as overvalued and underappreciated as cardiovascular physiology. The preoccupation with VO_2 max has detracted from the value of running economy, rendering it a misunderstood aspect of your running body. Science recognizes the value of being an economical runner and is able to correlate performance ability with running economy, but it doesn't quite know which training methods are best to improve it. As a result, running economy has become incidental to the training approach adopted by most runners—they train to improve VO_2 max, to develop their heart and lungs, to become better at using fuel to power the muscles; as a consequence, running economy invariably improves.

Perhaps we have reached the point where we should let go of preoccupation with VO_2 max and recognize that, in fact, it's economy of movement that determines your ceiling as a runner. We've described how speedwork, a deliberate focus on learning certain aspects of running technique, and training of the neuromuscular system through plyometrics and strength work might in fact produce bigger gains than the classically recommended training programs. That's not to say that running volume should be discarded and forgotten, because it's well recognized that running, like any other skill, improves with practice. So a good balance between building the base and incorporating special training sessions to improve economy is in order.

Chapter 6

Blood, Sweat, and Gatorade

You might think that as a runner, you have very little in common with a 250-pound NFL linebacker. But what you may not realize is that many of your beliefs and ideas regarding how much to drink when you run evolved out of the sport of football, and that your current beliefs on drinking were born out of research done on football players.

Specifically, in 1965 a Florida Gators football team assistant coach approached a Florida University kidney specialist named Robert Cade for advice about why players lost so much weight during practice. This initiated a research collaboration that would culminate in the creation of an entire sports drink industry and a specific product we all know as Gatorade, which has influenced science and knowledge perhaps more than any other in the field of sports science.

Cade and his team developed Gatorade as a result of research over a one-year period to discover why the football players were growing fatigued during practice sessions. That research found that the players tended to lose large volumes of sweat and that their blood sugar levels fell during the course of practice. Dehydration (from fluid lost in the form of sweat) and electrolyte loss (from sodium lost in the sweat) were identified as the causes of the problem. Cade developed a mixture of water, sodium, potassium, and some carbohydrates to replace energy and began providing it to the players during practice, and eventually during matches.

History records that the Gators improved steadily over the next few years, and they were particularly admired as a "second-half team" that became stronger and stronger as the match went on. When the Gators won the prestigious Orange Bowl in 1967, the losing coach's response to questions about why they had lost was, "We didn't have Gatorade. That made the difference." That is the kind of advertising money cannot buy, and Gatorade quickly became a sensation. It soon made its way into the professional ranks, where it gained a reputation as a miracle drink by all who used it. The early hype was such that widely read newspapers carried headlines like "One Lil' Swig of That Kickapoo Juice and Biff, Bam, Sock—It's Gators, 8-2" in 1966. The revolution in fluid replacement that began in football inevitably headed toward an explosion across all sports.

The running industry felt this explosion in a big way. Having come through the previous 60 years without the need for any product like Gatorade, runners were suddenly being told that the biggest dangers they faced were the threats of dehydration and of muscle cramps resulting from fluid and electrolyte loss. That explosion is the focus of this chapter.

Historical Beliefs of Runners: A Different Time and Different View

Had you been a runner at that time before the sports drink industry burst onto the scene, your attitude toward drinking would have been considerably different. You might, for example, have taken your inspiration from the great Jim Peters, who held the world record in the marathon event and once said,

"There is no need to take any solid food at all, and every effort should be made to do without liquid, as the moment food or drink is taken . . . some discomfort will almost invariably be felt."

Alternatively, you might have taken the advice of Jackie Meckler, a South African runner who won the grueling 90-kilometer Comrades ultramarathon five times, who said, "To run a complete marathon without any fluid replacement was regarded as the ultimate aim of most runners, and a test of their fitness."

Of course, we expect knowledge to evolve, and the advice of these great runners may have been completely incorrect and in need of revision. But it is interesting to note that the running fraternity had not seen any major need to investigate their fluid replacement strategies up to this point. Marathons were being run all the time, and no one had thought to question whether athletes were in mortal danger of illness or subpar performance as a result of not drinking more often. Quite why this is the case is a mystery—just as an NFL football player would lose fluid during training, typical marathon runners would be expected to lose perhaps 6 to 10 pounds during the course of the race, given that they were not drinking much at all.

Yet it was clear that these runners were finishing races in dreadful condition or slowing down dramatically at the end, perhaps because neither illness subpar performance was actually happening. Also, the actual incidence of dehydration with serious consequences was nonexistent. So running moved steadily forward without a major need to revise the generally accepted habits or beliefs. It took university football in Florida to drive that particular revolution.

Once the sports drink industry was born, however, that all changed. Over the course of the next 20 years, runners began to hear a very different message. Today they are instructed to avoid dehydration at all costs. Constant warnings are issued that any dehydration will impair performance; if it becomes severe enough, it will lead to heatstroke, a potentially deadly failure of the body to cope with increased heat production during running, and death. To prevent possibly catastrophic dehydration, the objective for runners should therefore be to start drinking early and then to drink often. Take, for example, the following advice, given to runners before one of the more popular marathons in 1996:

> DRINK BIG. Drink, drink, and drink some more. Not just on race day but every day. Dehydration is one of the most common causes of premature fatigue during training and competition, and it's also one of the most common causes of sports injuries—pulled muscles, cramps, dizziness, nausea, and heat exhaustion.

By this time, it's clear that not only had dehydration developed into a condition that could impair performance, but it was potentially responsible for just about any other problem that might occur during running, including cramps, which we'll tackle in the next chapter.

It was not enough to drink appropriately only during the race, and runners were encouraged to focus on practicing their drinking strategies during training as well:

> Like training for your big race, you need to train yourself to drink lots of fluids before, during, and after the race. Remember, practice makes perfect!

It is difficult to escape this message in the popular media—it is pervasive, aggressive, and ubiquitous and has become dogma among runners and exercise enthusiasts across all sports.

The Role of Science: Endorsement and Credibility

Science has been a major part of that marketing message. Gatorade was more than simply a sports drink—it spawned an entire research industry as well, and the creation of a Gatorade Sports Science Institute in 1985 confirmed a commitment to scientific research. Dr. Bob Murray, the former director of that institute, said, "Gatorade is the most researched drink on the planet," which it almost certainly is. Thousands of research papers have been published, many confirming that Gatorade helps performance, and no other commercial product has been as influential in driving research within the fields of sports medicine and exercise physiology.

In this regard, it's pertinent to question whether the lines between "scientific advice" and promotional strategy have blurred. A big part of the reason Gatorade is so widely researched is because Gatorade underwrites that research through its funding of scientists, laboratories, and its own institute. The obvious conflict of interest this creates is difficult to ignore, and while the research that was performed was often scientifically sound and credible, including well-conducted trials in controlled laboratory settings, the public interpretation and application of this research saw science become the endorser of the product. Just as companies spend millions so that celebrities will endorse their products, now privately funded science was positioned as a key driver of the marketing message that fluid intake was crucial and no athlete could do without it.

A Web site with a section dedicated to educating the public on fluid replacement needs, based on the Gatorade-funded science, is sponsored by the same company aiming to meet those needs. And perhaps not surprisingly, all the research of this period pointed in one direction—you need to drink, drink, drink.

Given the sheer weight of science behind Gatorade and the reported evidence confirming the dogma that dehydration is a potential killer, it's not difficult to appreciate why most runners believe that their fluid intake strategy will make or break their running. However, the marketing message that has been created around this scientific research creates an interesting dilemma when it is evaluated against what is actually happening to you, the runner, as you attempt to follow the advice (or ignore it altogether). In the giant laboratory that is the world of marathon running, for example, the observed facts and drinking practices are often completely irreconcilable with what has emerged from laboratory-based research.

A Black Swan in Fluid Intake: Reasons to Challenge the Paradigm

If we actually step back and evaluate the evidence, we might notice that elite athletes almost never drink the volumes they are "supposed to." For example, it is widely known that athletes who finish marathons in the fastest times are also those who lose the most weight. It could, in theory, be argued that if these runners drank more, they would finish even faster. However, this would create a huge problem in explaining why no one has figured this out yet. It would also mean that the world record in the marathon should be substantially faster because we know from our many interactions with elite runners that many who finish the marathon in 2:06 have lost up to eight pounds (or 5 percent of their body weight) during the run. Would they have improved their times by drinking an additional three liters of Gatorade? Even the most ardent supporter of the "drink big" philosophy would have difficulty arguing that one.

In this regard, today's elite athletes are not substantially different from those who ran marathons drinking very little fluid. Studies of elite athletes' fluid intakes during running, as well as self-reported strategies by these elite runners, have shown us that a fluid intake of about 200 milliliters per hour is typical. Given that these athletes are probably losing well over 1,000 milliliters per hour as sweat during running, according to the Gatorade-dehydration theory, they are headed for a problem.

So there seems to be a "black swan" in fluid-intake knowledge. Recall that we earlier defined a black swan as the single observation that renders all previous knowledge incorrect, a reference to the fact that people used to believe that only white swans existed. As soon as the first black swan was discovered, we had to reevaluate that entire position. So, too, we may need to reevaluate our position regarding fluid intake, dehydration, and body temperature regulation. That's not to say we'll throw out all that science because some of it is sound, but it's applying that information to you that we must discuss.

Finally, it's worth noting that the incidence of dehydration has not come down, but we have witnessed an explosion of another, far more serious medical condition, known as hyponatremia. This condition involves dilution of the blood to the degree that sodium levels fall, eventually affecting the balance of fluid across the cells. The consequences of fluid shifts in the body are catastrophic, leading to coma and death if left untreated. There has been a massive rise in hyponatremia cases, with several recorded deaths in recent years, and the adage that dehydration is the biggest threat faced by runners now needs revision—hyponatremia is a far more serious problem.

Perhaps it is time to reevaluate the position regarding fluid intake and running. But don't simply take our word for it—we'll unpack the research, the theories, and the concepts in much more detail in the coming sections, which will hopefully lead you to an improved understanding of just how much you should (or should not) drink when you run.

Theories of Dehydration

Clearly, something has changed in recent years, and depending on where you get your advice on what and how much to drink, the following might be familiar to you:

Never neglect the importance of hydration during marathon training. Even if it is cold outside and you don't feel like you sweat as much as if it were 90 degrees, you still need lots of fluid. You need to replace what you lose.

Fortunately many of the major marathons are moderating their hydration advice, but there are still many sources of information that tell you to drink, drink, and drink some more. It is important to understand why you are being told this.

For more than 40 years, dehydration, measured as a change in body weight during running, has been pegged as the reason behind everything from dry skin to decreased running performance to an elevated core temperature. It all started when Dr. John Greenleaf weighed subjects before exercise and then weighed them again right after they finished. During exercise, subjects were allowed free access to water, so they could drink as little or as much as they liked.

His main finding was that people do not replace 100 percent of their weight losses, which he took to equal fluid losses. In fact, the subjects in his study replaced, on average, less than 50 percent of their weight losses, and the term "voluntary dehydration" was coined to describe how humans choose not to replace all of our fluid losses during exercise.

The finding that people "dehydrate" laid the foundation for a number of assumptions and formed the basis for plenty of research over the past 40 years. That research, often funded by Gatorade, has been used to promote

theories, such as the one that says, "Dehydration of 2 percent causes performance to decline by 10 to 20 percent." This strikes fear into the heart of every runner, and the general response is to drink copious amounts of fluid in order to avoid this terrible condition at all costs.

Dehydration has also been blamed for increasing the core body temperature during exercise, which, you are told, causes you to collapse at the end of a race, and possibly even die. Performance and health are therefore both victims of this condition, which humans somehow choose to inflict on themselves, even when provided with unrestricted access to fluids. Because of voluntary dehydration, guidelines were developed to tell runners what they should do regarding the ingestion of fluid during exercise. These guidelines, which are brought out every decade or so by the American College of Sports Medicine, form the basis for much of the advice that is given through race Web sites, Internet sites, magazines, and running books.

The Influence of Dehydration on Health and Body Temperature

If you delve into the scientific literature, you will be hard pressed to find one single documented death from dehydration. Countless studies have shown that endurance athletes lose an average of 1 to 5 percent of their body weight during races, with some losing up to 8 percent of their starting weight. Yet these "severely dehydrated" athletes are never gravely ill. Most don't even enter the medical tent at races, in fact. Consider that the normal rate of admissions to the medical tent at races is about 1 percent of the starting field. Consider next that nearly everyone loses some weight during the race—the average value in marathon runners and Ironman triathletes is about 2 percent. We know from a number of published studies that there is no difference in the body weight change of athletes who collapse and have to be admitted for medical care and those who finish strongly and head home for postrace celebrations. This means that 99 percent of the field can be classified as having some degree of dehydration, yet they walk away from the race symptom-free. So fluid-related dangers during exercise do not involve drinking too little.

As far as your health goes, dehydration can affect the functioning of your cardiovascular system. You are, however, unlikely ever to experience this because fluids are readily available in American society, and generally we take in plenty of them when we eat our meals. Only in situations in which you're deprived of fluids will you experience any detrimental effects on your health. Yet you are

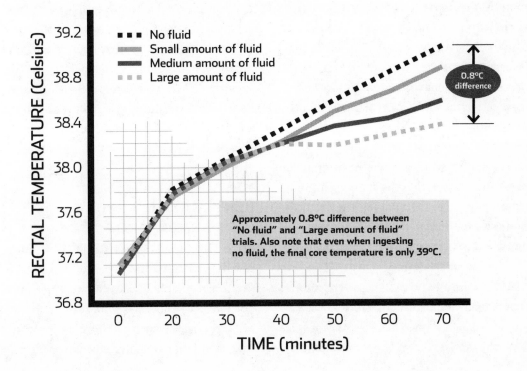

forewarned that failing to ingest sufficient fluids during exercise is a sure path to "heat illness," or even heatstroke. This has its origin in the lab. In 1970, Professor David Costill of Ball State University published the first study that investigated the effects of fluid ingestion on temperature regulation. He found that when runners ran at 70 percent of VO_2 max, at a sub-six-minute mile pace, and drank no fluid, their core temperatures were higher at the end of a two-hour run. As a result, the concept that the level of dehydration, as measured by weight loss during exercise, was responsible for driving core temperature higher during exercise was established.

We then move into the 1990s, which saw a more detailed variation of Costill's 1970 study. In this one, published in 1992 by Professor Ed Coyle of the University of Texas, cyclists cycled in a heat chamber for two hours while drinking different volumes of fluid. The title of this study says it all: *"The Influence of Graded Dehydration on Hyperthermia and Cardiovascular Drift during Exercise."*

The main finding, shown in the graph on page 101, is that when the cyclists drank no fluid (NF; the dark squares), they had the highest rectal temperature, and when they drank more (LF; the light squares), their temperatures were the lowest.

There were plenty of studies in the interim that helped support the findings of the two studies we have named here, but the message from the lab was clear: The amount of fluid you ingest will affect your core temperature. Specifically, if you do not replace 100 percent of your weight losses, then you will have a higher core temperature and thus be predisposed to heatstroke. This made risk reduction quite easy, as all one had to do was drink large volumes of fluid, and everything would be fine.

The Real Regulation of Core Temperature

Dehydration earned a bad reputation very early on, leading to advice from experts that may unwittingly have sparked the creation of a new, even more serious problem— hyponatremia, which we'll cover in more detail later. Fortunately, our bodies are a little more sophisticated than a car radiator system, and our understanding of body temperature regulation is a little more advanced. So let's discuss how body temperature is actually determined and set your mind at ease about the true influence of dehydration on body temperature.

METABOLIC RATE, NOT DEHYDRATION, PREDICTS CORE TEMPERATURE

Before the 1960s, you will not find much research on how fluid ingestion affects temperature regulation. The earliest thermoregulation study we know of is from 1938, performed by Marius Nielsen in Copenhagen and is titled "The Regulation of Body Temperature during

Muscular Work." Nielsen performed an exhaustive series of experiments on several men, in which he demonstrated that (1) the core temperature goes up as you exercise at higher power outputs and exercise therefore intensifies; and (2) core temperature is regulated at a higher level during exercise.

Fast-forward to 1963, when Sid Robinson published an article titled, "Temperature Regulation in Exercise." He began his summary of that paper with this:

> *The central body temperature of a man rises gradually during the first half hour of a period of work to a higher level, and this level is precisely maintained until the work is stopped ... During prolonged work, the temperature regulatory center in the hypothalamus appears to be reset at a level which is proportional to the intensity of the work, and this setting is independent of environmental temperature changes ranging from cold to moderately warm.*

Robinson's paper agreed with Nielsen's findings—namely that core temperature is regulated at a higher level during exercise. The point is that the body is quite happy with temperature change during running, and many variables are regulated at different (higher) set points when you run, without incurring problems. In addition, these scientists showed quite emphatically that metabolic rate determines body temperature. In other words, the harder you exercise, the hotter you become.

Until this point, little mention was made of fluid—it was all about work rate. Then the research on fluids we mentioned above was performed, changing everything. Now it was dehydration that caused body temperature to rise; gone were the roles of metabolic rate and exercise intensity. The science in those studies was good, but its application to your running races was wanting, for two reasons.

In the Costill study, elite-level runners (average VO_2 max of 74 ml/kg/min; including none other than *Runner's World* magazine editor at large Amby Burfoot) ran at speeds of about 9 miles per hour; the air blowing on them from a fan was moving at only 3.5 miles per hour, which is about the same as the speed of air when you're walking. Likewise, in the Coyle study, the cyclists were riding at power outputs corresponding to speeds of 20 miles per hour, yet the air moving over them was a breeze at a mere 6 miles per hour. If you have ever run outside on a cool day, you will be able to testify to the enormous cooling effect of a slight breeze. A strong wind on a cool day can make you very cold. Wind speed has a large impact on cooling potential. So in these studies:

→ Athletes exercised at a high intensity, which means that they were producing substantial heat; but ...

→ Their ability to lose that heat was greatly reduced, as they were denied appropriate wind speeds.

The lack of wind speed is crucial. Two of the coauthors of this book, Ross and Jonathan, published a study that repeated the famous Coyle study, except it used much higher wind speeds. It came as no surprise that when cyclists were provided with no wind, they could not even finish the two-hour trial, as they got too hot too quickly. On the other hand, when the wind speed was adjusted to match their power output, all of them finished the trial, and body temperature was unaffected by different levels of dehydration. Therefore, while the lab-based studies of Costill and Coyle showed a dehydration effect, it is arguable that this small effect was amplified by the lack of wind speed.

The other problem with lab studies is that scientists "fix" the power output. People do not exercise like this; in the real world we pace ourselves and speed up and slow down according to how we're feeling. If we slow down, our heat production goes down, and we do not get too hot. In the lab, the athletes are not allowed to do this, which is why we see a difference in core temperatures.

WHAT ACTUALLY HAPPENS: DATA FROM THE FIELD

Given that these lab-based studies are inappropriately applied to running races held outdoors, the solution to the dehydration problem has to come from studies that are actually

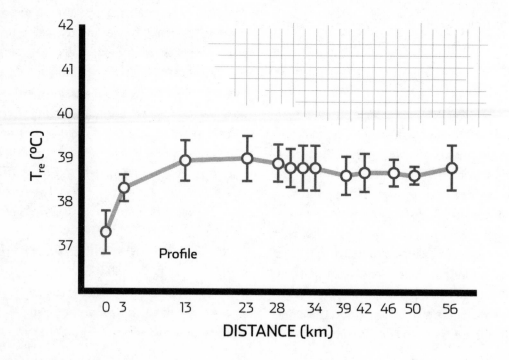

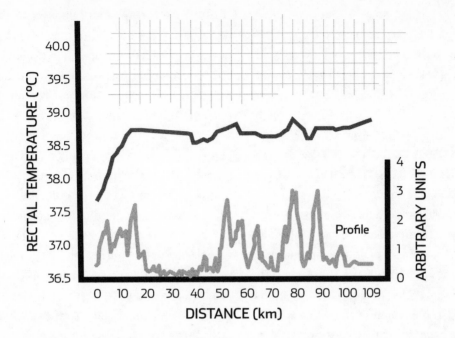

done in the field. Two studies from Jonathan's doctoral work measured the rectal temperatures of runners during a 56-kilometer race and cyclists during a 109-kilometer race. The main finding of these two studies was that the rectal temperature rises for approximately one hour and then levels off, after which time it remains within a very narrow range (less than 0.5° C). The data from the runners is on the opposite page, and the data from the cycle race is in the table above.

What both of these graphs show is that core temperature is maintained within a very narrow range during the event, which is not so different from what Marius Nielsen found 70 years ago. Secondly, most of the changes in core temperature occur *at the beginning of exer-* *cise,* rather than at the end. Thirdly, although the two groups were different—the runners were going simply for race completion and the cyclists were highly trained and racing— the temperature responses are similar. In addition, the environmental conditions were quite different in the two races: The weather for the marathon was cool and wet, and the cycling race was warm and dry. Yet the athlete's temperature response was similar, as was the amount of weight each group lost during their respective race.

These findings lead us back to the pre-1960s era, when the conclusion of scientists was that metabolic rate, or how hard you are exercising, is what determines your core temperature during exercise. Fluid does play a role, but the effect is small enough not to be meaningful. This means that ingesting large volumes of fluid is a waste of your time and raises the question of what, exactly, is the right amount?

Drinking according to the Dehydration Myth

If you follow the logic of the dehydration myth, then any amount of weight loss is bad. In fact, if you listen to Gatorade, you'll be told to replace 100 percent of your weight losses. The current guidelines from the American College of Sports Medicine call for a "customized fluid replacement program," which means you have to calculate your sweat losses and then design a program to match that volume. The latest version of these guidelines was released in 2007, a much-needed revision of the guidelines from 1996. The 1996 guidelines instructed athletes to avoid dehydration at all costs and to drink as much as tolerable during exercise. Runners often followed this advice to their detriment, because they usually exceeded their sweat rate (often by an enormous volume) and ended up gaining weight during the marathon and diluting their blood. This is a recipe for the development of hyponatremia, and the drastic rise in hyponatremia cases in marathon races in the 1990s was arguably a function of this advice given to runners.

Taking into account the growth of knowl-edge about and respect for hyponatremia, the latest guidelines have been toned down and now warn about drinking too much. They are still confusing, however, and do not offer much practical advice. Gone is the mantra to prevent all body weight losses; in its place is advice that says it is acceptable to lose up to 2 percent of your weight during exercise (but no more, by implication). However, the confusing part comes when the guidelines mention the extreme individuality of fluid needs during exercise and suggest ingesting moderate volumes of fluid *ad libitum*. The problem is that *ad libitum* means as much or as little as you like, and so qualifying this advice with a volume is problematic and confusing. Practically, this advice fails, because a plan is only as good as the conditions it's worked out for, and so the target of losing less than 2 percent of your body weight is nearly impossible to hit with any accuracy.

More significantly, the dissemination of new information to the public is slow, and so the general perception of coaches, athletes, and the public remains that dehydration is to be avoided at all costs. Coaches, athletes, magazine authors, and even medical doctors repeat the same message: Drink to prevent body weight losses. This is no doubt because Gatorade still advocates that athletes replace 100 percent of their weight losses, and the power of marketing trumps that of scientists publishing recommendations in scientific journals.

Drinking according to Common Sense: Obey Your Thirst!

In physiology, we often talk about how a particular variable is regulated, or "defended," as the body activates mechanisms to keep some substance within a particular range or value. The marketing messages we're exposed to tell us that when it comes to balancing fluid in our bodies, body weight is the relevant variable. But this does not make sense, because your body actively allows you to lose weight during running, and there are no other systems in the body that we must "tell" to do otherwise in order to survive and keep functioning.

The consequence of this focus on body weight is that you have been led to believe that thirst is a poor guide to your fluid needs. This "thirst is bad" concept stuck because of the power of marketing and advertising, and a mantra was born: "If you wait until you're thirsty, it's too late." The dehydration paradigm places body weight ahead of fluid in the "physiological pecking order" of what is important to regulate.

Physiologically, however, the reality is that humans (and all other mammals) have very well developed and successful mechanisms in place to help conserve and maintain fluid balance. The body is not concerned about body weight but instead about the concentration of the body's fluids, otherwise known as *osmolality*. Here is how it works.

Incredibly small increases (1 percent) above the resting value first will trigger the release of *antidiuretic hormone*, or ADH. Its job is to keep you from losing any more water in urine. It has a profound effect; even small amounts of ADH produce a maximal effect—that is, once ADH is secreted, it is not possible for you to produce any less urine. Next, if ADH does not do the trick, as is the case when you're exercising and sweating, thirst kicks in. Again, this occurs at a very marginal (4 percent or less) elevation of osmolality. The effect is that we seek fluid and drink it; eventually the fluid reaches the blood and dilutes it below the thirst threshold. This cycle continues indefinitely until you stop excreting fluid (i.e., sweating) and restore your osmolality, at least until your next run.

In fact, humans have a very acute sense of when it is important to drink fluids, and it does not take much to stimulate us to seek water. Thirst is a very deep-seated, physiological desire for water, and it has been shown again and again in lab studies to effectively defend osmolality, not body weight.

The reason the body does not regulate weight losses and instead defends osmolality is that this concentration of body fluids is what maintains the fluid balance between cells. There is fluid both inside and outside our cells, and under normal conditions, osmolality maintains this balance. The following two changes are possible:

→ The osmolality can increase outside the cells. This will cause the fluid to leave the cells. Because this is undesirable, the ADH and thirst mechanisms described above kick in, and we correct the change to restore balance.

→ The osmolality can decrease outside the cells. If this happens, then fluid will move into the cells. Similarly, the body will initiate a sequence of responses, including the release of other hormones (aldosterone, for example) that eventually address this change, returning osmolality to normal and making sure that fluid stays in the appropriate cellular compartments.

Because our bodies are mostly water, you can imagine why keeping these fluid volumes balanced is so important. That is precisely why the body defends osmolality and not body weight. And when you drink to regulate body weight, only trouble can occur, as you are now second-guessing your body and eons of physiological evolution.

So if there is one thing you remember from this chapter, or indeed this book, let it be that your thirst mechanism is one of the most sensitive, well-developed, and exquisite mechanisms you have. If you simply obey it, you will never run into any dangers with dehydration or heatstroke. Therefore, drink according to thirst, no more, no less, and you will optimize both performance and health. However, if you try to balance fluids based on a formula,

attempting to calculate your sweat rate based on weighing yourself before and after a run, the risk is that you may exceed that rate during a race. If that happens, then you run a very serious risk of hyponatremia.

The Biggest Danger of Fluid during Exercise— Hyponatremia

Ignoring your degree of thirst and drinking to a schedule is a sure way to overload the body with fluid. There is a delicate balance of the fluid inside and outside the cells. If we overload the fluid outside, sodium concentration in the blood falls, producing the condition called hyponatremia. When this happens, fluid will shift inside the cells, which is a problem, especially in the skull, as your brain is very sensitive to changes in pressure.

Since 1986 there have been numerous cases of hospitalization following running events, and unfortunately several have resulted in death. The cause of these unfortunate events is not dehydration, however, but the exact opposite: drinking too much fluid. When you drink more than your body weight changes and thirst levels dictate, you run the risk of developing hyponatremia.

What Hyponatremia Is Not

Although this condition describes a low sodium concentration in the blood, it may surprise you that hyponatremia is not a sodium imbalance in your body. People have tried to attribute hyponatremia to the excessive loss of sodium in sweat, but this is incorrect, because although there is some sodium in sweat, compared with the fluid in your body it is a low concentration. Therefore, when you lose sweat, it actually causes the concentration of sodium in your blood to rise, and this triggers you to drink fluids to bring it back down. So although you lose some sodium when you sweat, this does not cause hyponatremia.

What Hyponatremia Is

Based on the explanation of what hyponatremia is not, you might be able to use some deduction and figure out what it is. If you said hyponatremia is a problem of fluid balance, you would be correct. As you add fluid—either water or a sports drink—in quantities greater than you would consume if you were drinking according to thirst, it causes your sodium concentration to drop. Why is this? When we sweat, we remove some of the fluid volume and leave most of the sodium behind, but when we ingest too much fluid, we add a dilute solution to our blood, which will inevitably cause the sodium concentration to fall. Consider a simple comparison: mixing a sports drink from a powder. If you scoop the required amount to make a half gallon into a jug and add just one cup of water, of course you will have a very concentrated drink. If you add the amount the directions call for, then you have the optimal concentration for that drink. However, if you continue to add water to that drink, it becomes diluted. The same thing happens in your blood when you ingest more fluid than you would when using thirst as your guide.

I Think I Drank Too Much . . . What Do I Do?

Many athletes we speak to tell us that they do not know when they are thirsty, and they insist that they need a prescribed set of rules for fluid ingestion. While it may be hard to believe that runners know when they're thirsty, we can offer this: In nearly every race, someone overdoes it and ends up in the medical tent, often having gained weight thanks to fluid overload and then developed potentially fatal hyponatremia. Here is how to identify the problem and what to do about it.

SIGNS AND SYMPTOMS: ASYMPTOMATIC HYPONATREMIA

The typical signs of a mild fluid overload are headache, nausea, and bloating. In addition, the runner's watch or rings might be very tight, because there will be some swelling in the arms and legs. The problem is that headache and nausea are also signs of dehydration. The sure way to differentiate between the two

Drinking Too Much Can Kill You

The first reported case of hyponatremia in the scientific literature was in 1986. It was a runner in the 90 kilometer Comrades Marathon in South Africa. The woman was in grave condition and was hospitalized; ultimately she recovered. There were other cases over the years, but the first known death from hyponatremia during a running event occurred in 1998.

Kelly Barrett was running the Chicago Marathon that year when she stopped just a mile from the finish. Paramedics picked her up and, believing her to be dehydrated, reflexively administered IV fluids. After just four ounces, Barrett stopped breathing. She survived long enough to be admitted to the hospital, but, sadly, she died three days later—her brain had been damaged when she stopped breathing, and the function never returned. This was an incredible tragedy because it was so preventable, but surely runners would learn from this rare but powerful event.

Yet, four years later, in the 2002 Boston Marathon, the tragedy played out once again. This time it was another young woman, Cynthia Lucero, who collapsed around mile 20 and was taken to the hospital in an ambulance. Unlike Barrett, though, Lucero never made it to the hospital and died on the way. According to the friends supporting her on the course, Lucero drank large amounts of Gatorade, and the undeniable lesson from her case is that even sports drinks can cause hyponatremia, although Gatorade still claims that drinking its product will prevent the deadly condition.

Unfortunately the story does not end here, and cases of hyponatremia continue to appear. Just a few months after Lucero's death, it was another woman at the Marine Corps Marathon, and in 2007, a runner in the London Marathon was hospitalized and died from drinking too much. Every race at which the authors have worked has produced at least one case of nonfatal but severe hyponatremia.

Bottom line: Drink according to thirst, as it will always prevent you from drinking too little, and, more important, it will prevent you from drinking too much—which can be fatal.

vastly different conditions is bloating and swelling. Also, if you're throwing up large amounts of fluid, you cannot possibly be dehydrated. By definition, dehydration means no fluid left. We often see athletes who are vomiting almost pure water. If you or a friend experiences these symptoms, report to the medical tent immediately and let the staff know that you might have ingested too much fluid during the event.

SIGNS AND SYMPTOMS: SYMPTOMATIC HYPONATREMIA

If the condition is a bit worse, the symptoms become progressively graver. Vomiting will almost surely be present, and you will appear to be "not all there." The technical term is *altered mental status*, and it means that the swelling is affecting the brain and causing some mental dysfunction. The runner probably will not know where he or she is, what day it is, or even who you, a friend, or family member, are. If someone you know has these symptoms, go immediately to the emergency room or the medical tent, whichever is closer. This condition may worsen at any moment; seizures might develop. If the sodium concentration is low enough, then perhaps respiratory arrest, coma, and eventually death could follow.

Our aim is not to scare you, but you must understand that the real danger when it comes to fluid replacement during exercise is not from drinking too little but from drinking too much. Remember that there are no documented deaths from dehydration but several from hyponatremia.

TREATING THE PROBLEM

If your condition is severe enough, you will not have a hand in your own treatment, and it will be left to the sports physician. If you do notice that you have some swelling and are bloated and nauseated, however, then the one thing you must not do is ingest any more fluid. You are not dehydrated. Drinking more fluid will only make the problem worse, and you might end up in the hospital. Instead, stop drinking fluids. Eventually you should begin to pass large volumes of very dilute urine. However, if you do not urinate within 24 hours after the finish of your race, go to the hospital. You might be experiencing acute renal failure, especially after an ultramarathon, which produces significant amounts of muscle damage.

Chapter 7

The Mysterious Muscle Cramp

In the previous chapter, we discussed the physiology of body temperature and fluid regulation during exercise and suggested that drinking according to thirst is more than adequate to meet your fluid needs when running. That advice is quite different from the messages you'll encounter in magazines and media advertising, which tell you that any level of dehydration is dangerous and could cause impaired performance, hyperthermia, and even death. What makes the "danger and death from dehydration" message so convincing is that it is almost always backed up by men in white lab coats with letters behind their names and by research studies that seem to prove that dehydration is dangerous. This research is often taken out of context and wrongly applied; there is just as much, if not more, research that shows that dehydration is not dangerous. Instead, it's drinking too much that you need to fear. The body's exquisite thirst mechanism is perfectly able to tell you when and how much to drink, and you can do a lot worse than simply "obey your thirst," as a very different sort of advertising message commands.

In this chapter, we turn our attention to muscle cramps, which have also been caught up in the marketing mythology of dehydration and fluid loss. Muscle cramping, with a lifetime prevalence of more than 50 percent, is perhaps the most common affliction that affects runners. Most runners, particularly those who run marathons, will at some stage in their running careers experience cramping. If you have never cramped, then count yourself lucky—you are part of the distinct minority.

Defining Cramp and Explaining Its Occurrence

A cramp is somewhat laboriously defined as a *"spasmodic, painful, involuntary contraction of the skeletal muscle that occurs during or immediately after exercise."* Note that this definition applies to exercise-related cramps only, and therefore it excludes a whole host of other categories of cramps. Other cramping that occurs outside of exercise may be symptomatic of a hormonal, neurologic, or vascular disorder or may be caused by certain drugs or occupational factors. Then there are cramps that are what the experts call idiopathic, which technically means they have no cause (but in reality means doctors don't know what causes them). If you regularly experience cramps, either during exercise or when at rest, it's probably worth seeing a doctor to determine whether any of these broad factors might be responsible.

As for exercise-associated muscle cramps, the cause remains poorly understood and highly controversial, with two conflicting theories being the source of much debate among scientists. One of these theories is that cramps are caused by fluid and electrolyte loss, which has therefore been the focus of much Gatorade-sponsored research. It is thanks to this research that runners are frequently warned that "dehydration is one of the most common causes of premature fatigue during training and competition, and it's also one of the most common causes of sports injuries—pulled muscles, cramps, dizziness, nausea, and heat exhaustion."

It doesn't end there. A trip to a local pharmacy or sports shop to glance at the seemingly infinite number of supplements, gels, drinks, creams, and other products that are designed to prevent cramps will help you realize that just as the dehydration theory of overheating and exercise fatigue spawned an industry, so too have muscle cramps driven an industry of their own, aided and abetted by scientific research with sometimes questionable motives.

Let's evaluate the prevailing theory critically and see if we can't arrive at a more likely explanation for exercise-related muscle cramps and, with it, some better ideas about how to prevent them.

A BRIEF HISTORY OF CRAMPING: THE ELECTROLYTE DEPLETION THEORY

The earliest theories about muscle cramping date back more than 100 years, when laborers in the hot and humid conditions of mines and shipyards suffered from cramps. Even that far back, it was possible to analyze sweat, and it was observed that the cramping workers had a high chloride level in their sweat. (Chloride, incidentally, is half of the salt in your sweat. Sodium, which we shall meet shortly, is the other half.) The theory back then was that in hot and humid working conditions, excessive loss of fluid and electrolytes caused the muscles (and nerves) to malfunction, resulting in cramps. Later, the builders of the Hoover Dam recovered from cramps when they drank salty milk, entrenching the theory that salt loss was the cause of cramping.

These two anecdotes form the basis for the theory that is widely held as true today: Cramps are caused by excessive loss of sodium and chloride in sweat. Later, calcium and magnesium were added to the mix, and heat and humidity were implicated as "accessories." The term *heat cramps* became an alternative name for muscle cramps associated with activity. This is particularly interesting, because in the Hoover Dam study, it was found that not a single cramping worker had a body temperature above 38.5°C (101°F), so heat was actually dismissed as a cause of cramps more than 70 years ago. Somewhere between then and now, however, it regained its foothold and has today become deep-rooted.

An important point about the Hoover Dam research is that no one measured the sweat content of the laborers who *did not cramp*, and so whether their electrolyte levels were different from those of the cramping workers is not known. Also, cramping laborers were immediately removed from their work positions and brought to the surface or allowed to rest while they drank their milk, leaving open the possibility that it was the act of

working that caused the cramp, and simple rest alleviated it, regardless of what the workers drank during that rest.

Nevertheless, it became an accepted fact that fluid and electrolyte depletion, combined with high body temperature, cause exercise-associated muscle cramps. As a result, it has become dogma that dehydration is to blame for cramping and that drinking is the cure, as shown by the following expert testimonies:

→ When a young athlete experiences heat cramps, pull him or her off the field into a cool area and gently stretch the affected muscle. Have them drink, drink, drink, and then drink more," says Albert C. Hergenroeder, a professor of pediatrics at Baylor College of Medicine and chief of the sports medicine clinic at Texas Children's Hospital.

→ "High-sodium drinks will prevent children from getting heat cramps," says Jackie Berning, PhD, of the National Alliance for Youth Sports. "Gatorade has just enough sodium to prevent those cramps. But if you're a heavy sweater, and you're still getting cramps after drinking Gatorade, eat some salted pretzels or salted nuts. Those work fine."

Muscle cramps and dehydration are now inextricably linked, not only regarding potential causes but also in terms of how research has been used to entrench perceptions and drive sales of products to prevent them. (The second quote in particular, a very thinly veiled promotional pitch for Gatorade, is similar in nature to what we described previously as "scientific endorsement" of products regarding fluids.) Of course, there is nothing wrong with this in principle—scientific innovation should drive product development; witness the entire history of the pharmaceutical industry. The problem is that the scientific evidence is often contrary to what is popularly reported, and it does not back up the expert opinions, including those discussed earlier.

DEHYDRATION UNDER THE SPOTLIGHT

The dehydration theory of cramping should be quite simple to evaluate and prove. All it requires is that you collect a group of athletes who experience cramps, plus a control group of athletes who seldom or never cramp, and put them all through a hot, sweaty workout. You should be able to show that:

→ The athletes who cramp are more dehydrated than the noncramping athletes.

→ The cramping athletes have reduced blood electrolyte concentrations compared with the noncramping athletes.

A simple descriptive study of this sort would go a long way toward confirming the hypothesis, and then it might be possible to further define the mechanism. However, you may be surprised to know that this simple study has never been performed, and in fact, the opposite has been found—runners who cramp tend to have lost less weight (i.e., are less dehydrated) and have electrolyte levels similar to those who do not cramp. We'll consider those studies now.

LABORATORY VERSUS FIELD RESEARCH: OBSERVING WHAT REALLY HAPPENS

Perhaps the greatest problem affecting our understanding of muscle cramps is that no one has yet created a laboratory protocol in which scientists can deliberately induce muscle cramps in a controlled, reliable manner. It is impossible to predict with certainty when cramping will occur, so controlled laboratory studies of athletes in which their fluid intake and electrolyte levels are systematically measured have been impossible to perform.

The alternative is a field study, in which athletes are observed during their typical exercise activity and analyzed only after the event. These studies are often descriptive in nature, and force scientists to work backward to attempt to identify a possible cause.

FIELD STUDIES: DEHYDRATION AND ELECTROLYTE LOSS ARE NOT THE CAUSE

Field studies have brought out some very interesting findings, not least of all because they punch some sizable holes in the dehydration theory of muscle cramps. Recall that if a muscle cramp is caused by dehydration and electrolyte loss, then runners who cramp should have low electrolyte levels and a greater level of dehydration (measured, typically, as body weight loss during the event). However, two large-scale studies have found the exact opposite—runners who cramp are less dehydrated and have electrolyte levels that are normal and similar to those of a noncramping control group.

In the first of these two studies, published in 2004, Martin Schwellnus of the University of Cape Town and his colleagues examined runners before and after the 56-kilometer Two Oceans Marathon. Their main finding was that when crampers were compared with the controls (who were matched for body mass and finishing time), the only differences were that the crampers had *lower* sodium levels and *higher* magnesium levels. Neither value would be considered abnormal, however. In fact, the crampers, with a value of 139.8 mM, had a textbook sodium concentration—no doctor would be concerned by a patient whose sodium level was near 140 mM.

	Crampers (N = 21)	Controls (N = 22)
Sodium (mM)	139.8 ffl 2.1*	142.3 ffl 2.1
Potassium (mM)	4.9 ffl 0.6	4.7 ffl 0.5
Magnesium (mM)	0.73 ffl 0.1*	0.67 ffl 0.1
Osmolality (mM)	280 ffl 6	284 ffl 10
Body weight change (% loss)	2.9 ffl 1.2*	3.6 ffl 1.2

What is also noteworthy from this study is that the crampers had an average body weight loss of 2.9 percent, compared with 3.6 percent for the noncramping controls. In other words, the people who cramped actually lost *less weight* than noncrampers, indicating that a greater level of dehydration had little to do with cramping. This, combined with the slightly lower (though still normal) sodium levels, suggests that overhydration, not dehydration, characterizes people with cramps.

There's more to it than this because Schwellnus was also able to measure the change in plasma volume—a more direct measure of what is happening to body fluids. He found that the crampers actually increased their plasma volume by 0.2 percent during the race. The noncramping control subjects *lost* 0.7 percent. By any interpretation, this data was the wrong way around. It was not, however, a once-off finding because one year later, Schwellnus took the same concept to the Ironman triathlon, and his findings were remarkably similar.

The Ironman triathlon, consisting of 2.4 miles of swimming, 112 miles of cycling, and a standard 26.2-mile marathon to the finish, is one event in which the loss of electrolytes and fluid must surely be a major factor. After all, it takes the winners more than 8 hours to finish, and most finish in more than 12 hours. Given this extreme race duration, an Ironman triathlete loses many liters of fluid and many grams of salt between the starting line and the finish line, so the event is the perfect "laboratory" in which to evaluate whether dehydration and electrolyte loss drive muscle cramps.

Schwellnus's data are again surprising but repeat the pattern observed in the Two Oceans Marathon:

	Crampers (N = 11)	Controls (N = 9)
Age (years)	33.5 ± 8.8	35.4 ± 8.1
Prerace mass (kg)	79.1 ± 5.9	77.7 ± 6.4
Postrace mass (kg)	76.3 ± 5.6	74.6 ± 6.5
Body mass loss (%)	3.4 ± 1.3	3.9 ± 2.0
Total race time (min)	660.8 ± 77.9	685.7 ± 48.5

As was the case at Two Oceans, the crampers actually lost less weight than the noncramping athletes in the Ironman triathlon. Looking at their electrolyte levels, it's again clear that the cramping athletes had normal sodium, potassium, and magnesium levels.

	Crampers (N = 11)	Controls (N = 9)
Sodium	140 ± 2	143 ± 3
Potassium	4.4 ± 0.06	4.2 ± 0.5
Magnesium	0.9 ± 0.2	0.8 ± 0.1

Given the dogma surrounding muscle cramps and electrolytes, it is difficult to know how this information can be interpreted. It clearly demonstrates that something is wrong with the theory that athletes who cramp are dehydrated, with abnormally low sodium levels. They may indeed lose sodium in their sweat, as has been shown to occur in studies on football and tennis players, but what is happening in the body is quite different—cramping runners are physiologically indistinguishable from noncramping runners, apart from the unexpected finding that they are less dehydrated. The value of drinking sports drinks and taking electrolyte supplements to prevent cramps becomes an open question.

THE PROBLEMS WITH THE SERUM ELECTROLYTE DEPLETION THEORY: SWEATING INCREASES SODIUM CONCENTRATION

In addition to the data suggesting a flawed theory, there is also a significant conceptual problem with the theory that dehydration causes cramps. This concept, ignored by advocates of a fluid-based model for cramping, is that when

Sweating and Your Sodium Levels

To see how sweating causes electrolyte levels to rise, imagine you have five cups of water and five teaspoons of salt. If you remove one cup and one teaspoon, the balance remains the same—there is one spoonful of salt for every one cup of water (a concentration of 1.0).

However, if you remove one spoonful of salt and two cups of water, you can see that the number of spoons relative to cups has increased—you have lost more water than salt, and the concentration of salt has risen as a result (to 1.25). Now, imagine that you mix all these spoonfuls of salt into the water and perform the same exercise. As soon as you remove more fluid than salt (as happens when you sweat), you are in effect "straining" your salt-and-water mixture and creating a new, much saltier solution.

Applying this concept to physiology, we know that the sodium concentration of blood is about 140 mM (put differently, this means that there are 3.2 grams of salt for every one liter of blood). Your sweat, on the other hand, has a sodium concentration of about 20 to 50 mM. This value varies widely, as we'll see when we discuss "salty sweaters," who apparently have high sodium levels, but the average is probably about 50 mM. This means that you lose about 1.1 grams of salt in every liter of sweat.

Given the difference between your blood and your sweat, it's clear that you lose more fluid than sodium when you sweat, so your sodium concentration will actually rise as you become more dehydrated. This is a crucial conceptual point, because the theory that cramping is caused by low electrolytes as a result of sweating cannot be true if the act of sweating cannot possibly lower your electrolyte concentration.

you sweat, you do not actually reduce your body's electrolyte concentration—you increase it. There certainly are electrolytes in the sweat, but the concentration of them is so low compared with the concentration of electrolytes in the blood that sweating will only increase electrolyte concentration in the blood. We say that the sweat is *hypotonic* (meaning its electrolyte concentration is low relative to that of blood plasma), and the result of sweating is that your blood becomes *hypertonic* (more concentrated than normal). Of course, the total amount of electrolytes (the absolute mass of sodium, for example) decreases, but this has never been pointed to as the cause of muscle cramps. Only hypotonicity has, and again, sweating makes the blood hypertonic, not hypotonic (see the box above).

This theory is borne out by studies of runners taking part in marathons and ultramarathons. Most runners are observed to have lost some weight (usually about 2 to 3 percent of their starting body mass) and have slightly elevated blood sodium levels by the time they reach the finish line. They are what we call *hypernatremic,* as opposed to those runners who become hyponatremic as a result of drinking too much water. We (Jonathan and Ross) have worked in the medical tent of the Comrades ultramarathon in South Africa for the past three years, and 80 percent of the finishers we saw lost weight and had high sodium concentrations. It's clear-cut: Fluid loss does not cause sodium concentration to fall; it causes hypernatremia. This, of course, poses a major problem for the theory that salt loss and dehydration cause cramping. In order to overcome this problem, one would have to find people who lose an abnormally high amount of sodium in their sweat. This group is called the "salty sweaters."

SALTY SWEATERS: A CREATED GROUP OF THE POPULATION THAT STILL FAILS TO EXPLAIN THE THEORETICAL OUTCOME OF SWEATING

"Salty sweater" is the term applied to a person who has a very high salt concentration in his or her sweat. Many Web sites and popular magazines are now issuing warnings to all "salty sweaters" to take extra care to replace their salt and prevent dehydration during exercise, by eating pretzels, for example. There is a problem, however: No one actually knows what a salty sweater is. How much salt does there need to be in the sweat before you qualify for this group? No one knows. Recently, Professor Schwellnus, widely published in this area, posed this question to scientists at the Gatorade Sports Science Institute at a conference on cramping. He received no answer.

We might, for the sake of argument, assume that a "normal" sodium content of sweat is 50 mM. This is actually on the high side; most runners have much lower levels than this. However, let's assume that salty sweaters have 100 mM of sodium in their sweat. This is a very high value and should satisfy any definition of a salty sweater. This person loses 2.3 grams of sodium in each liter of sweat. However, remember that the sodium content of the plasma is 3.2 grams per liter, so it is immediately obvious that even a salty sweater will experience an increase in blood sodium when he or she sweats, because more fluid is lost than sodium, relative to the plasma. Only when the sodium content of sweat exceeds 140 mM (which hasn't been documented in field studies) does a theoretical problem even begin to exist.

So, apart from the fact that no one really knows what a salty sweater is, the saltiest sweaters still have hypotonic sweat—the more they sweat, the more their electrolyte levels rise. This point also has implications for how you replace the sodium you lose during exercise. The sports drinks that you may believe help with sodium replenishment are in fact ineffective, because they, too, are hypotonic and only dilute the plasma further (see page 125).

Surprisingly (or perhaps expectedly, given the commercial incentives to promote the theory that dehydration causes cramps), both the research and this concept have been all but ignored in the field of sports science. Few runners are ever told of it, and advocates of the dehydration-electrolyte theory never respond to these challenges. This information most certainly is not featured on any Web site giving people advice on how to prevent cramps. As a result, we have no explanation for how an athlete with normal electrolyte levels and less fluid loss can experience cramps. It would seem to be time to describe an alternative hypothesis, a model for how cramps might occur in the absence of dehydration or electrolyte loss.

AN ALTERNATIVE HYPOTHESIS FOR MUSCLE CRAMP: FATIGUE AND A REFLEX GONE WRONG

The alternative theory has its origins in a paper published in 1997 by Martin Schwellnus, whom we introduced earlier in Chapter 3 as the scientist who found no association between electrolyte levels and cramp risk in runners and Ironman triathletes. His alternative hypothesis was that muscle cramps were the result of dysfunctional reflex control of the motor nerve as a result of fatigue. That sounds like a mouthful, but we'll pull it apart piece by piece.

A good way to start is to ask a few pointed questions about muscle cramps. Those readers who've experienced them (more than half of you reading this, no doubt) will know the answers to these questions instantly, but they are important pointers to help understand the cause of cramping.

Q. *Which muscles are most likely to cramp?*

A. This is a pretty important question. The answer, of course, is the active muscles. Few runners have ever cramped in their arms, and if they have, then this is probably a far more serious problem than we typically recognize or speak about as exercise-associated muscle cramp; people suffering from hyponatremia, for example, can experience generalized cramping (and this, you'll recall, is a problem caused by drinking *too much*). The fact that only the active muscles cramp (quads, hamstrings, and calves in runners) points toward a mechanism that is associated with the act of muscle contraction as a possible cause of cramp. We have already seen that there is no association between electrolyte levels and cramping risk.

Q. *What is the most effective treatment for a cramp?*

A. Apart from stopping (and, often, collapsing), the most effective thing you can do for a cramping muscle is to stretch it, as you no doubt know intuitively. You also know that if you try to contract the muscle, or shorten it, you make the problem far worse. If you experience a cramp in your calf muscle, for example, and you try to point your toe away from your body, you will find yourself in instant agony. The question is why? Something associated with stretching the muscle helps prevent cramp, while contracting it only makes things worse. Our alternative explanation must account for this fact.

Q. When is cramping most likely to occur?

A. There is evidence that muscle cramps happen during racing and not training. They also tend to happen nearer the end of races. One could of course argue that it's only at the end that the electrolyte levels drop to the point where they cause cramps, but again, we've seen that crampers have very normal electrolyte levels. Also, a long training run is just as likely to cause fluid and electrolyte loss, yet cramping is less likely to occur in this context, so something associated with racing is responsible. Studies have also found that racing on a course that is hillier than an athlete's normal training grounds and racing above a level of training that can be comfortably handled are predictive factors for muscle cramps. That is, people who cramp are invariably racing harder or starting a race at a faster pace than their training has prepared them to do.

These three questions introduce some important points that are not easily explained by a simple electrolyte depletion model. A plausible theory of exercise-associated muscle cramps must explain why cramping occurs at normal electrolyte and hydration levels, why only active muscles cramp, why stretching a muscle is the most effective treatment, and why muscles typically cramp in circumstances of extreme exertion. In order to do this, we first have to appreciate the basics of the neural control of muscle activity.

The Normal Reflex Control of Muscle Function

Your muscles are stimulated to contract by a group of nerves known as *alpha motor neurons*. When you perform any motor task (touching your finger to your nose, running, and so forth), a signal from the motor cortex of the brain travels down the spinal cord, leaves the spinal cord, and travels to the muscle fiber along the motor nerve. Once at the muscle, the electrical signal being delivered is responsible for muscle contraction (by way of a process we covered in Chapter 1).

There are other pathways that also affect movement; of course, it's not as simple as a single impulse traveling down the spinal cord to the muscle. The complexity of a simple motor task such as placing your finger on your nose is absolutely astonishing, and it involves many other brain areas and muscle groups. But for our purposes, what is important is that when alpha motor neuron activity increases, the muscle contracts. We must now consider the factors that cause alpha motor neuron activity to increase. There are three pathways that can activate the motor neuron and thus cause muscle contraction:

→ First, there is the higher central control we described above.

→ Second, there are spinal interneurons.

→ Third, and most important for our cramp discussion, the alpha motor neuron is also regulated by what is called spinal reflex activity; there are two particular reflexes that need to be addressed.

The Muscle Spindle Reflex

You've probably heard of or experienced the classic knee-jerk reflex, when a doctor (or a friend) taps on your knee tendon with a small hammer and you can't help but kick out with your foot. That simple test demonstrates the first important reflex.

The muscle spindle is a tiny structure in each muscle fiber, and its job is to make sure that the muscle does not stretch too much. Every time your muscle is stretched, muscle spindle activity increases. This sends a signal back to the spinal cord (along what are called Type Ia afferent nerves), where the nerve impulse is passed on to the alpha motor neuron, activating it and causing the muscle to contract. In other words, when you stretch the muscle, the reflex response initiated will cause the muscle to contract—a protective action that prevents overstretching of the muscle.

Now, referring again to the knee-jerk reflex, tapping on the knee causes your quadriceps muscle to stretch. As a result, the spindle fires, Type Ia afferent activity to the spinal cord increases, and then alpha motor neuron activity increases. When the alpha motor neuron fires, it causes the *same* muscle to contract, and that is why your quadriceps contracts and your leg kicks out in response.

The key point here is that if the muscle spindle firing rates go up, then the muscle will contract.

The Golgi Tendon Organ Reflex

The second reflex that influences muscle activity is called the Golgi tendon organ reflex. The Golgi tendon organ performs a very different role from that of muscle spindles; it monitors the tension in the muscles and tendons, rather than the stretch. It is active when the muscle is contracted or lengthened, which puts load on the tendons. Its role is to make sure that the muscle does not contract too forcefully or under too much load. When the muscle is placed under load (any contraction), the Golgi tendon organ fires, and it sends a signal to the spinal cord along what is called a Type Ib afferent.

This time, however, a key difference is that Type Ib afferents tell the alpha motor neurons to stop firing—the Type Ib afferents are inhibitory. So, when the Golgi tendon organ fires, then the alpha motor neuron activity decreases. This reflex causes a reduction in muscle contraction. The effect, of course, is again protective, because it prevents the muscle from taking on too much load. If you have ever tried to pick up a very heavy weight and found that you suddenly lose all strength and have to drop the weight, then you've fallen victim to the reflex protection of your Golgi tendon organ.

The take-home message this time is that if the Golgi tendon organ is stimulated, the end result is that muscle contraction is switched off. However, if the Golgi tendon organ is inhibited, then alpha motor neuron activity will increase, and the muscle will contract even more—this is called *disinhibition*.

SO WHAT HAPPENS DURING RUNNING, AND CAN IT EXPLAIN CRAMPING?

In studies of muscle function and fatigue, the following have been found:

→ When muscle becomes fatigued, the firing rate of the Type Ia afferent fibers from the muscle spindle increases.

→ The firing rate from the Type Ib afferent fibers from the Golgi tendon organ decreases.

The effect of fatigue will therefore be to activate the alpha motor neuron on both counts—increased firing from the muscle spindle and decreased firing from the Golgi

tendon organs both contribute to an increase in the firing rate of the alpha motor neuron.

You will recall that when the alpha motor neuron fires, the muscle contracts, so fatigue will cause an involuntary, reflex contraction of the muscle. This theory places fatigue, not electrolyte depletion or dehydration, as the central cause of muscle cramps. It says that fatigue interferes with the normal control of the muscle, and an involuntary, reflex contraction is the result.

There is evidence that this is the case. The electrical activity of the muscles of cramping runners was measured after the Two Oceans Marathon, and it was found that the alpha motor neuron activity was higher than in noncramping athletes. Because of the previously mentioned difficulty in creating a study that induces muscle cramps in the laboratory, research has proven elusive, and further evidence is needed to either confirm or refute the theory. Ideally, science needs a study that induces cramps in athletes while measuring both their electrolyte levels and the electrical activity in the muscle throughout exercise to definitively prove or disprove either hypothesis.

This fatigue-based theory does, however, explain the questions we posed earlier in this chapter:

Q. *Which muscles are most likely to cramp?*
A. The active muscles cramp because they are, in this alternative model, the source of the

problem, since their fatigue is the cause of the reflex dysfunction. Research studies have found that if you experimentally lower electrolyte levels, or if they are lowered by overdrinking, generalized cramping occurs. An electrolyte theory for cramping therefore predicts cramps in both active and inactive muscles.

An extension of this explanation is that the muscles that are most likely to cramp are those that cross two joints, such as the calf muscle (which crosses both the ankle and the knee joint). Without going into an anatomy lesson, these kinds of muscles have to contract while they are in a shortened position. Think of when you are swimming, for example, and your toe is pointed down, so your calf contracts in that shortened position. The shortened position of the muscle means that the Golgi tendon organs are unloaded, so the situation is perfect for cramp to occur if the muscle spindles start to fire with fatigue. This is why calf cramps, especially in swimming, are so common.

Q. *What is the most effective treatment for cramp?*

A. The most effective treatment for muscle cramps is passive stretching, as any athlete knows. A passive stretch is known to gradually lead to a reduction in the firing rate of the muscle spindle and an increase in the rate of firing from the Golgi tendon organs. As explained, these changes will eventually reduce the firing rate of the alpha motor neuron, causing muscle relaxation. At first, however,

putting the muscle into a stretched position is extremely painful, because the initial stretch causes the spindle firing rate to increase. This is why the poor cramping athlete often gets worse before he or she starts getting better. However, over time the spindle firing rate decreases, and the cramp is eventually alleviated.

Q. *When is cramp most likely to occur?*

A. The fatigue-based model explains why cramping is most likely to occur during races, rather than training, and why studies have found that tough, hilly courses and poor pacing are also predictive of muscle cramps.

In the electrolyte theory, one would also expect cramps to occur toward the later stages of exercise, so this is not as convincing as other lines of evidence. But nevertheless, every cramper has experienced the disappointment of successfully putting in three or four hours of training, only to find that three hours of racing causes a cramp. Also, athletes often cramp during relatively short-duration exercise, when there simply is not enough time to deplete the electrolytes. (And keep in mind that we have explained that this concept of electrolyte depletion through sweating is false.) Finally, the finding that cramping occurs on hilly courses also suggests that fatigue is a key component in the muscle cramp story.

Sports Drinks: An Ineffective Method of Replacing Sodium

Sports drinks are incapable of defending the body's sodium levels during exercise, despite what the manufacturers and advertisers tell you. The sports drink industry has created the perception that its electrolytes will help prevent a decrease in sodium. (Recall the expert testimony we presented earlier: *"Gatorade has just enough sodium to prevent those cramps."*) This is incorrect for two reasons. First, sweating does not cause a drop in sodium to begin with—it causes an increase, as we have explained. And second, sports drinks contain insufficient sodium to counteract the effects of sweating on the blood's electrolyte concentration, and in fact cause the sodium level to fall further.

Why? Because a sports drink contains approximately 18 mM of sodium, or only 0.4 gram of sodium per liter. This means that if you drank one liter of Gatorade during exercise, you would replace a full liter of fluid but only 0.4 gram of sodium. Recall that blood normally has 1.4 grams of sodium per liter, which means that even a sports drink replaces more water relative to salt and will only lower your sodium concentration.

If, for example, you were to drink three liters of Gatorade while reading this chapter, your blood sodium level would fall by approximately 5 mM, to 135 mM (supposing that a few assumptions we make in doing the necessary calculation are accurate). As this hypothetical example illustrates, you cannot elevate or defend your sodium levels by drinking a sports drink. It is impossible.

Having said that, we must add that if the alternative is water, then sports drinks do help prevent the sodium level from falling as much as it might. In other words, if you are going to drink as much as you can, then a sports drink will cause a smaller decline in sodium than water will. The key point is that sports drinks still cause a decline, but less than that caused by water. The act of drinking is still what ultimately causes the reduction. The impact of the sports drink is also tiny—approximately 2 mM over the course of a two-hour event.

In consideration of this reality, Gatorade advocates consuming additional salt by eating pretzels or salty snacks. Again, this advice is fundamentally flawed, because unless you're drinking too much, you don't need to supplement with sodium. It's a case of two wrongs trying to make a right and, it has to be said, more money. You're better off not overdrinking in the first place. Just listen to your thirst (and hunger), and obey what it suggests you do.

PREVENTING CRAMPS: APPLYING THEORY TO PERFORMANCE

We have presented two models for the cause of cramps. The first model attempts to explain them based on electrolyte disturbances and dehydration. The second model is based on the effects of fatigue on neural activity and muscle excitation and relaxation. So which one is correct?

The short answer is that we do not know exactly what causes cramps, and it will probably be many years (perhaps even decades) before someone presents a more definitive model that better explains their cause. It's fairly clear that there are some major flaws in the electrolyte model, which is not supported even by measurements of electrolytes in crampers compared with noncrampers. Conceptually, and based on data, the electrolyte model is full of holes. The fatigue model is, however, incomplete, lacking the data to either support or disprove the proposed sequence of events.

The bottom line is that it is a complicated mechanism, like so many other physiological phenomena. Also, just as our many different physiological systems are affected by a vast array of factors and circumstances, it's likely that cramping is the result of the interaction of many factors. Until we have a reliable laboratory protocol that can reproduce cramps in a predictable manner, we cannot really test the models further. For now, we can begin to make some suggestions for how one might prevent cramps based on the fatigue model.

Cramp Prevention the Fatigue-Model Way

To begin with, there is a strong likelihood that cramping has a genetic component, in that some runners are predisposed to cramping. Quite what this gene is or how its impact can be negated is as yet unknown. However, there are a few strategies that all runners can adopt to reduce the likelihood of cramping, regardless of their starting risk.

First of all, given that the reflex dysfunction is probably caused by fatigue, anything you can do to prevent muscle fatigue should help prevent cramps. This is why runners often find that they can handle long training runs, yet shorter-length races cause severe cramps—the difference is the higher intensity of the race, leading to fatigue. The obvious, though undesirable, avoidance strategy, then, is to simply slow down. A survey of Ironman athletes in South Africa found that it was possible to predict who would cramp based on an analysis of the athlete's personal bests coming in and his expressed goal time. That is, athletes who had a goal time that far exceeded what their historical performances suggested they were capable of were more likely to cramp. This is because these athletes would start out at a pace that was simply too fast for their physiology, leading to premature fatigue.

Therefore, knowing your own abilities is key, as it will help you select the right pace from the outset of your race. There is little doubt that cramps are more likely to happen in athletes who start too fast. The difficult part is defining what "too fast" means, and that's best left to the individual.

Second, a stronger muscle is likely to resist fatigue, so your training should focus on developing strength in susceptible muscles. Some runners know that they cramp in the calves, others in the quads, others in the hamstrings. Specific strength training may help to prevent the reflex dysfunction, and regular crampers should seriously consider adding a well-designed strength component to their training.

In addition, there is no substitute for strength work that is running-specific. Hill training, speedwork, and sufficient long runs are crucial elements of a complete program. This is especially important if you are preparing for a race that you know has hills or will push you to your limit due to extreme distance or some other factor. The groundwork is laid in training, so don't leave these elements out; preparation and training are the keys to hitting the starting line with a minimal chance of cramping.

Regular stretching may also help reduce the incidence of cramping. As we've already explained, stretching is an effective means of treating cramps because it reduces the alpha motor neuron activity. But stretching before the cramp occurs (if you are susceptible) may help prevent this dysfunction from occurring. Again, this is speculative, since no laboratory protocol exists to induce cramps; therefore, preventive measures such as stretching cannot be evaluated in studies. However, there is little to lose (apart from a few seconds) in trying preventive stretching, so our advice is to stretch during the event before you cramp. At regular intervals at water tables and aid stations, it may help to lightly stretch the muscles you know are predisposed to cramps.

Finally, what of the various remedies and products available to prevent cramp? Many athletes swear by electrolyte gels or salt tablets as cramp-preventing agents. The data from field studies don't support this effect, since crampers and noncrampers have similar electrolyte levels. Also, for every athlete who finds that electrolyte supplements work, there are probably five who take them and cramp anyway. No study has ever shown their effectiveness, and even the anecdotal evidence is quite weak.

However, some athletes perceive that it works, and sometimes perception is reality. Therefore, if you are one of those who swear by salt tablets, then don't fix what is already working for you. We can't argue with those who say, "Who cares if it can't be proven, provided it works?" It may be a placebo effect; it may be a sign of something that is not yet explainable. After all, as we said at the outset of this chapter, cramps, despite their high prevalence, remain something of a mystery, and no absolute answers exist.

PART 3

The Metabolic

System

If the muscles are the pistons of the runner's body and the cardiorespiratory system is its engine, then the metabolic system is the fuel that powers it. The most fatigue-resistant muscle in the world, the highest VO_2 max or best running economy on the planet, and all the training in the world are rendered completely meaningless if the metabolic system fails to do its job of providing the energy required to enable all those processes to happen. Any runner who has experienced the dreaded bonk, when they suddenly find their blood glucose levels falling as a result of insufficient energy intake, will testify to that fact.

Metabolism also creates one of the body's most amazing processes—a story of enzymes, chemicals, reactions, and products that is ultimately responsible for allowing you to run. The premise of the metabolic system is pretty basic: Your active muscle, and every other organ in your body, needs ATP—the accepted energy currency throughout the body. But we don't store ATP in the muscles and organs. That would be biochemically impractical. Instead, we store energy in the form of carbohydrates, fats, and, to a lesser extent, proteins. These macronutrients are stored in muscle tissue as well as in the liver (carbohydrates), and adipose tissue (fats), until they are required by the active muscles during exercise.

As soon as we start running, the story begins. A complex set of reactions takes place to break down these storage forms of carbohydrates, fats, and proteins and convert them into usable forms, which are then broken down further, to result in the formation of ATP. This story has innumerable characters, many of which are no doubt familiar to you, though perhaps not in the roles in which you'll see them in this section.

First, there are the hormones, which kickstart the process by switching on enzymes, the drivers of the metabolic reactions that produce ATP. Adrenaline, your body's fight-or-flight hormone, which is released in times of stress (like when you begin running), is one such messenger. It acts in the liver, the adipose tissue, and the muscle to switch on the breakdown of carbohydrates and fats. The enzymes it switches on convert carbohydrates into glucose and fats into fatty acids. Glucose and fatty acids then undergo a series of controlled, step-by-step reactions (which are a nightmare to every undergraduate biochemistry and physiology student) that ultimately result in the production of ATP.

Our focus is not to understand these reactions or to explain how certain enzymes are switched on while others are switched off. Those are details we'll allow the body to take care of. We're interested in how we can tap into the processes to find ways to help improve your running performance. Not surprisingly because of the crucial role of energy provision during exercise, science has focused heavily on the metabolic system as a crucial limitation to performance. ATP depletion, glycogen depletion, and lactate accumulation have all been identified, studied and implicated as possible contributors to fatigue. Experienced marathon runners the world over warn of "hitting the wall," the dreaded point at which the body's muscles and liver run out of glycogen. We can delay fatigue, the theory goes, by finding ways to use less carbohydrate and more fat. Those ways include diet, both before and after the race; certain supplements; and, of course, training.

The metabolic system provides one of the most profound reasons why endurance training works: It enhances your body's fuel system by helping you store more energy, use it more efficiently, and supply energy to muscle in greater quantities and at greater rates. It's all about supply and demand—training increases supply. All in all, understanding how carbohydrates and fats are converted into ATP will go a long way toward making you a better runner.

Then there is what you put into your body. The metabolic reactions taking place in the muscle are only half of the equation. First you must supply energy to the body, providing the fuel before you train and while you train. What are the best foods during training and races? What is the best postexercise meal? Understand metabolism, and you'll appreciate the answers to these questions.

We also address the issue of habitual diet, which has implications for health as well as running. When your body is not using carbohydrates and fats for energy, it's in storage mode—and storage usually means fat. Obesity and its related health problems are reaching pandemic proportions, but as a runner, you may have managed to steer clear of that minefield. Or perhaps you're a runner because you happened to enter it. Regardless, you'll benefit from knowing what to eat, healthwise as well as runningwise.

[Chapter 8]

Maximum Fuel Economy

If you knew that tomorrow morning you'd wake up and leave for a road trip across the USA on the famous Route 66, one of the first things you would do in anticipation is drive down to your local gas station and fill up your car's tank. You'd do this, of course, because you recognize that without energy, you'll go nowhere. Once under way, you'd also pay close attention to road-side signs indicating distances to the next fuel stop because you know that few things will spoil your journey like an empty fuel tank somewhere between Albuquerque and Oklahoma City. Of course, in this day and age, the chances of this happening are slim, as hardly 15 minutes pass between potential fuel stops.

Let's now say that instead of a trip along Route 66, you're planning a series of long runs in preparation for your next race. These runs are going to last between 2 and 4 hours each (anything less would be considered a short journey, for which fuel supply is not as crucial, as we'll see). If you are prudent, one of the first things that will come to mind as you plan these runs is fuel—where do you get it during the run, and how do you fill your "tank" before you start? It's likely that most of you will recognize that the physiological equivalent of running out of gas is not a pleasant experience—it's called "hitting the wall," or "bonking," which sounds more like a head-on collision than a gradual grinding to a halt, and with good reason. To allow you to run long distances, strategies to make the most of your fuel are as important as the training you do.

Energy Supply during Exercise

We've already seen that running economy—the use of oxygen at submaximal running speeds—may be an important determinant of endurance running success. But equally important, and occasionally more important, is your ability to use your fuel stores to produce ATP as effectively as possible. As we've seen in previous chapters, the production of ATP from the body's carbohydrate and fat stores is crucial to allow muscle contraction to continue. In short, depletion of energy means the lights go out.

Every runner has either heard of or experienced what is colloquially called the bonk. It happens when the level of glucose in the blood falls very low, the result of the depletion of glycogen stores in the liver and muscles.

Glucose is stored in the liver and muscles as glycogen and is used during exercise; we replenish it when we eat. The liver is particularly important in this regard because it is responsible for releasing glucose into the blood and is therefore the key player in maintaining the blood glucose concentration within the correct range. Glucose release is triggered by any stress, including exercise, that causes the hormone adrenaline to be released. Before you even start running, the body has already anticipated it and released adrenaline into the blood.

Adrenaline does its work in both the liver and the muscle, breaking down glycogen to form glucose. In muscle, glucose is used for energy production, whereas in the liver, glucose is released into the blood so that your muscles and all other tissues, including the brain, that are using up ATP are able to replace it and keep you going.

The brain also uses some of this glucose, but unlike the muscle and the heart, which can use fat for fuel, the brain relies on glucose for its energy supply. This is why depletion of liver glycogen and the resulting drop in blood glucose concentration cause the symptoms you may have experienced on long runs when you failed to ingest sufficient carbohydrate: light-headedness, fatigue, tunnel vision, nausea, loss of coordination, and an overwhelming desire to stop running. Often, the most spectacular (and somewhat morbid) images of long-distance runners "failing" are those of runners staggering toward the finish line, clearly hitting the wall on every stride. These symptoms illustrate the dramatic effects of low blood glucose levels. By the time this "dance of the headless monkey" occurs, you can imagine the muscles are struggling to produce their own energy.

So it is crucial for runners to manage the availability of carbohydrates when they exercise, especially over long distances. To complicate matters further, bear in mind that the body is not restricted to using only glycogen and glucose for energy production. There are two additional sources of energy:

→ Fat stored inside the muscle, or intramuscular triglycerides. Like muscle glycogen, this store is available for immediate use within the exercising muscle.

→ Fat stored in fat cells, known as adipose tissue, located all over the body. The use of this energy store is somewhat more complex because the fat must first be broken down into molecules called fatty acids. These fatty acids must then be transported from the adipose tissue into the muscle. A complex series of reactions, pathways, and enzymes exists to make this happen, which we won't spend too much time on, other than to say that the challenge of using fat as fuel lies in delivering fatty acids to the muscle in a usable form.

Protein is an additional source of energy which we won't spend too much time on, either because it becomes a factor only in very severe cases, such as ultraendurance exercise or when energy intake is severely restricted, as in the case of starvation. In all other circumstances, protein is broken down to amino acids during exercise, but these amino acids are rapidly reconstituted after exercise, provided adequate protein is consumed between runs. In other words, it's only when the run-ner fails to replace energy that the circulating amino acids are converted to glucose and contribute to energy production, resulting in net protein loss. Obviously, the longer or more extreme the exercise bout, the more difficult it is to ensure that this balance is maintained. That's why ultraendurance athletes, especially adventure racers, multiday marathon runners, and extreme runners, have to pay close attention to postrace diet. However, since we're talking more about pre- and in-race energy here, protein won't figure as heavily as fats and carbohydrates.

Making the Most of Fuel Stores

With regard to how fuel use holds the key to performance, there are perhaps three key points to understand. The first has already been described: When the body's muscle and (especially) liver glycogen stores are depleted, exercise becomes impossible. You have to either stop altogether or slow to a walk. This process is regulated by the brain so that you never reach complete depletion. In this regard, it's subtly different from the earlier car analogy; if the gas tank becomes bone dry, the engine actually stops running. Your body never completely runs out of carbohydrates, and there is evidence that individual athletes have "off switches" that engage at different levels of depletion. But in every athlete, that "off switch" engages at relatively low muscle glycogen and blood glucose levels, so if you wish to maximize performance, you must do what you can to minimize the decrease in blood glucose and muscle glycogen.

The second key point is recognizing that the carbohydrate stores—liver and muscle glycogen—are limited in size and volume. Even with optimal training and diet, you might be able to "pack" about 200 grams of glycogen into your liver and up to 500 grams into the muscle. That's good enough to keep you going for around two hours, which is why "hitting the wall" usually happens after 20 miles—the duration required to deplete glycogen stores. Interestingly, while you sleep, your brain uses up the glycogen in the liver, so you wake up in a nearly liver-glycogen-depleted state, which means a run first thing in the morning is going to be even more challenging. Often, even 45 minutes may prove too much in such an early morning run, unless you're accustomed to it, as we'll see.

On the other hand, the stores of fat (muscle triglyceride and adipose fat) are virtually limitless (much to the dismay of many, no doubt!). For example, 176-pound man with a body fat percentage of 16 percent (normal value) has almost 29 pounds of fat, equating to 26 tubs of margarine, and while it isn't all usable, it's clearly more abundant than the paltry 600 grams of carbohydrate.

The third key point is that any adaptation you can make in the following three areas will almost surely result in improved endurance performance:

1. Maximize your stores of carbohydrates before you start running.

2. Reduce your body's reliance on stored carbohydrates during the run, thereby delaying their depletion.

3. Increase the reliance on fat stores when running, so that you spare the body's carbohydrate stores.

These three goals of training and fueling for endurance have driven much of the strategy, research, and thinking about training and diet in recent years, and they form the basis for discussion in the remainder of this section.

1. HOW CAN YOU MAXIMIZE CARBOHYDRATE STORES BEFORE YOU START?

The answer to this one is fairly well understood and is practiced by runners the world over. It involves the physiological equivalent of filling the tank before the journey starts. In runner-speak, it's called *carbo-loading*, which usually involves a few days of increased carbohydrate intake before the race.

The scientific understanding of carbo-loading and performance took off in the 1970s, driven by the development of a technique called muscle biopsy, which allowed researchers to take a piece of muscle from an athlete and measure how it had changed during exercise. Not an altogether pleasant experience for the runner, but the information gained by actually looking inside the muscle helped scientists figure out how fuel was being used. It was during this time that the first evidence emerged that carbo-loading could improve performance by delaying the drop in muscle and liver glycogen levels and thus fatigue. This finding has been replicated in a number of studies, though there are a couple of conceptual problems with and limitations to the methods used, which we'll discuss shortly. However, the general consensus, which persists to this day, is that runners doing long-distance training or racing should do their level best to take in as much carbohydrate as possible before the event.

Most long-distance runners take this advice to heart, but whether they actually take it to their stomachs is another question. Recent evidence suggests that despite their best efforts, athletes often undereat and fail to take in the right amount of carbohydrates. Two keys to successful carbo-loading are the amount and the timing of carbohydrate intake; 40 years of research and testing provided the following answers to these questions:

How much?
The optimal range is between 10 and 12 grams per kilogram per day. So, for an 176-pound

(80-kilogram) runner, we're talking 800 to 900 grams per day. The box on page 149 shows the amounts of typical foods that contain 50 grams of carbohydrates. It's quite clear from this list that carbo-loading to the recommended level is no mean feat. For example, if you ate only baked beans, you'd need 16 to 20 cups per day. That is, by any standards, a tall order—and not one that we'd recommend for a very pleasant race experience.

Obviously, you won't restrict your carbohydrate intake to only one source, so throughout the day, you're likely to take in close to 500 grams quite naturally. The balance is perhaps easiest provided through commercially available carbo-loading drinks and powders, mixed with either milk or water. Drinks are good because they provide a concentrated source of carbohydrate, which is needed when you're aiming as high as this.

What's the best process and timing?
There was a time when the recommended strategy was to first deplete your body's carbohydrate stores by not eating much for a couple of days and then carbo-load. Scientists noticed that after the depletion phase, the body responded by compensating and actually storing more than it would have before. However, it was soon realized that athletes, who are effectively depleting their stores just by training, don't need to follow this practice. Instead, three days of high-

carbohydrate foods combined with reduced training (as one would typically do before a race) is enough to cause the same "supercompensation" effect.

Carbo-Loading versus a High-Carbohydrate Diet for Training

Given the volume of food required, it's perhaps not surprising that many people fall short of the optimum when it comes to carbo-loading practices. Of perhaps greater concern for endurance runners is that the habitual diet followed by runners is often nowhere near the level required to replace the energy they use on a day-to-day basis. This is not directly relevant to carbo-loading but is no less crucial. For example, if you run an hour a day, you need to take in roughly 5 to 6 grams of carbohydrate per kilogram of body weight. If you are more serious and train two hours a day, then your daily requirement goes up to 8 to 9 grams per kilogram. For an 176-pound (80-kilogram) man, that is around 650 grams a day, a target that requires a concerted effort to reach, even with a big appetite.

Recently, a new area of research has looked at low-carb diets and their effect on performance. In these studies, athletes are given a restricted diet during their training periods, with the aim of seeing how the body adapts and how performance might be affected by training with minimal carbohydrate. It turns out that when the athlete finally does take in some carbohydrate, performance actually improves. It's likely that runners are doing their daily training with severely limited energy stores and adapting to this restriction. When they are finally provided with more fuel, the brain senses this, and runners' perceptions of effort are greatly reduced. It's the physiological equivalent of a banquet feast after months of semistarvation. Of course, this practice is not recommended, and you're far better off aiming to meet the optimal needs from day one, even if it means consulting a dietitian for specific advice on which foods are best for you.

But Does Carbo-Loading Actually Work?

The early evidence for carbo-loading was very positive. Numerous studies found that if athletes were carbo-loaded, they could exercise longer before voluntarily calling it quits; this improvement was associated with a higher starting glycogen level in the muscles and liver and with a longer time before blood glucose levels dropped below normal, signifying liver glycogen depletion.

However, these studies were always somewhat contrived. For one thing, they measured performance simply as "time to fatigue" at a fixed work rate. That is, runners or cyclists exercised at the same pace until exhaustion—hardly representative of the way you run a marathon. There have been some studies that have shown that when the athlete can slow down or speed up, the performance advantage of carbo-loading is not nearly as clear.

Secondly, these studies often use cycling, a non-weight-bearing exercise, in a laboratory as the exercise trial. The situation is quite different as soon as you have to do a weight-bearing activity because carbo-loading causes substantial weight gain. It is not uncommon to gain 7 to 9 pounds in the final three days before a race, thanks to the storage of extra glycogen and the water stored with it. Many runners would jump at the chance to run 7 to 9 pounds lighter, so there's some question as to whether the benefit of additional fuel that comes with carbo-loading is offset by the detriment of weight gain.

The third point is that these studies usually deny access to carbohydrates during exercise. The athlete is instead forced to rely on his or her starting carbohydrate stores and nothing else. This is analogous to embarking on your Route 66 road trip without any possibility of stopping along the way for gas. Clearly, that's not a realistic prospect, since you have the option of providing energy throughout your runs. In the past three decades of carbohydrate research, it has been proven that providing energy continuously during running largely diminishes the value of topping off the prerun stores, as we'll see in the next section.

Finally, none of these studies have investigated carbohydrate metabolism and loading control for any placebo effect. The placebo effect is well known and understood in any experiment when subjects are given some kind of treatment or intervention. For example, even in clinical drug trials, some of the subjects in the placebo group, who are receiving an entirely inert pill, will report improvements in their condition. The improvements are not limited to subjective measurements, either, and oftentimes the physiological variables are also different.

There are two major challenges when trying to control for the placebo effect in carbohydrate loading studies. The first is that when you put someone on either their normal diet or a carbo-loading diet, it is quite obvious which diet they are on, as it is difficult to mask an additional 200-plus grams of carbohydrate a day. Second, runners the world over undoubtedly know the "rule" that you must carbo-load before the marathon to enhance performance, and so there is a clear bias among the subjects in the studies.

For these reasons, carbo-loading is likely to be ineffective, possibly even detrimental, to performance in events shorter than about two hours. A half-marathon athlete need not concern himself with carbo-loading—the added weight is inhibitive and access to energy on the run sufficient. For longer runs, we'd still recommend a high-carbohydrate diet leading up to the race, but it is probably more important to ensure that the day-to-day diet is up to standard. The final three days are much less important than the three months before them. The diagram on page 150 summarizes the effect of carbohydrate intake on fuel sources and also provides guidelines for the carbo-loading phase and the crucial training diet.

2. HOW CAN YOU REDUCE YOUR BODY'S RELIANCE ON CARBOHYDRATE STORES TO DELAY FATIGUE?

Once the race or training run has actually started, the next strategy is to delay fatigue by reducing the rate at which glycogen from the liver and muscles is used. This can be achieved by taking in carbohydrates during the run. Energy replacement during the run is crucial to success in long-distance events. Most runners can recount tales of trying to complete a long-distance event without any form of carbohydrate consumption and the disastrous consequences they experienced.

Taking in carbohydrates while running is beneficial for two reasons. First, it provides yet another source of glucose to the muscles and brain, which helps maintain the supply of energy to meet the increased demand. The second reason is that drinking or eating carbohydrates during exercise effectively provides the liver with a "crutch" during exertion and defers some of the pressure to maintain the blood glucose concentration.

Recall that the liver breaks down its glycogen into glucose and releases the glucose into the blood. If you are able to supply that glucose from another source (a sports drink, for example), then the liver doesn't need to put out as much glucose. The result is that liver glycogen is spared, and you can run longer before hypoglycemia develops. In scientific terms, we say that *exogenous* (meaning from the outside) glucose supply supplements the body's *endogenous* (internally stored) supply.

Interestingly enough, ingesting carbohydrates doesn't make much impact on the use of muscle glycogen—it's as though this fuel store is "locked away," and the muscles will use what they have available regardless of whether other supply sources are at hand. However, the impact on liver glycogen is large, especially in the latter phases of exercise; after hours of running, the glucose gained from your sports drink becomes crucial. So there are good reasons to make use of the sugary drinks provided along the route of your next race.

The question is how to optimize this energy replacement. There are three key characteristics of the ideal energy replacement strategy:

Content: What should you drink?

In terms of what to drink, the scientific evidence suggests that basic sugars, which are absorbed rapidly into the blood for immediate use, are ideal. The glycemic index is not important during your race. This means that glucose, maltose, and maltodextrin are ideal. Maltodextrins are glucose chains found in most energy gels and some sports drinks. Gatorade and Powerade contain glucose, which is the most basic sugar unit. The only "bad" sugar during exercise is fructose because it must first be converted to glucose in order to be used for energy production, and it can also cause stomach problems during exercise. Interestingly, when fructose is mixed with other sugars, this problem does not seem to be an issue. Recent studies have shown that sports drinks containing fructose and glucose supply carbohydrate to the muscles faster than sports drinks that contain an equal amount of carbohydrate in the form of glucose alone, precisely because the body metabolizes the two sugars through two completely separate channels.

Most commercially available energy products contain the optimal *types* of carbohydrates, but what is more important is their *concentration* of carbs. Too low, and you provide the body with far less than optimal energy to sustain exercise. If too high, first you will struggle to empty the drink from your stomach; when you eventually do, water is actually pulled into the intestine by the highly concentrated mix. Absorption is impaired, and digestive problems such as diarrhea can occur.

Research suggests that the optimal concentration is between 6 and 9 grams of glucose per 4 ounces of product (6 to 9 percent). If you take a look at a bottle of Powerade sports drink, for example, you'll see that it contains 7.8 grams of carbohydrates per 100 milliliters, which is right in this range. The gels are somewhat more varied, containing anywhere between 15 and 25 grams per packet. The onus is obviously on you to make sure you dilute them correctly. If you are taking one full packet containing 20 grams, for example, then you need to drink about 9 ounces of water with it in order to get the desired 8 percent concentration. Many runners fail to do this and therefore end up either with a sugary blob sitting in their stomach or with digestion trouble. So take care to ensure that you get the dilution right—know how many grams you're ingesting and then drink enough water to speed the process of emptying your stomach and the rate of intestinal absorption.

Amount: How much do you need?
The amount of energy required depends largely on your running speed. The faster you run, of course, the more glucose you'll use. But the fastest running speeds cannot be sustained long enough for glycogen depletion and hypoglycemia to limit performance. These factors come into play only during runs lasting hours, in which the running speed is

likely to be relatively low. Given this fact, the amount of exogenous, or external, carbohydrate you need per hour ranges between 50 and 60 grams.

Considering that your optimal concentration is about 8 percent, if you are getting your glucose from a sports drink, about 20 ounces per hour will suffice. If you use a gel, then a 20-gram packet every 25 minutes does the trick, along with 9 ounces of water. It's not too difficult to meet this requirement, which is a somewhat conservative one.

Timing: When should you drink it?

The timing is dictated partly by the required amount. If you need 50 grams per hour and your drink contains 8 grams per 4 ounces, then you need about 16 ounces of the drink per hour, which can be achieved in any number of ways. For example, you could drink all 16 ounces every 60 minutes, if you wished. Studies have found, however, that the best results come with high frequency fluid intake. In other words, drink small amounts often: 16 ounces per hour is best achieved as 4 ounces every 15 minutes. This approach not only avoids the bloating you'd feel if you suddenly drank 16 ounces, but also supplies fluid and glucose to your bloodstream faster.

It's important to begin energy replacement soon after the run begins—within the first 30 minutes is recommended. In very long events (ultramarathons) lasting upward

of 8 hours, it's common that the continual ingestion of these sugary drinks either causes nausea, or else you just get so sick of the taste after several hours that you would rather go without than try to choke down another cupful. In these cases, you should realize that you can't consume only energy gels for 10 hours. Plan ahead. Consider bananas, potatoes, pretzels, sandwiches, energy bars, or any other type of carbohydrate you have access to and can tolerate. In addition, it might help to try savory foods to break the monotony of sweet sports drinks and gels.

The figure on page 151 summarizes the physiological effects of carbohydrate ingestion during exercise and the recommended strategy for consuming carbs on the run.

3. HOW CAN YOU INCREASE YOUR BODY'S RELIANCE ON FAT STORES WHEN RUNNING?

The third and final avenue for performance improvement is perhaps the most intriguing and widely researched strategy today. Whereas carbo-loading and carbohydrate ingestion have been studied for 40 years and are quite well understood, the use of fat during exercise is still something of a mystery.

The principle is the same, however: If your body can be taught or forced to use more fat, then the carbohydrate stores are spared and fatigue will be delayed. As we saw earlier, the body's virtually limitless supply of fat makes it an extremely attractive fuel option for those wishing to achieve maximum fuel economy during running.

There are many strategies for increasing the body's reliance on fat during running, but we'll focus on two of these:

1. Endurance training
2. High-fat diets (fat-loading)

Endurance Training: Teaching Your Body to Be a Fat-Burner

For the long-distance runner, one of the most important adaptations to training is the ability to use more fat at a given running speed. In other words, before training, a runner going at, say, an eight-minute mile pace will get perhaps 50 percent of his energy from glycogen stores and 50 percent from fat. Six months later, with perhaps 500 miles of running training behind him, this ratio will have changed to 40 percent from carbohydrates and 60 percent from fat. A heavier reliance on fat means less reliance on blood glucose and muscle glycogen, and that means delayed fatigue and improved running performance.

This adaptation is quite complex in nature and involves enzymes, pathways, transporters, and hormonal adaptations, which we won't go into. The bottom line is that training increases the capacity of the muscles to use fat. Recall that the main fat store in the body is adipose tissue. In order to provide energy in the muscle, this fat must first be:

→ Converted to a fatty acid molecule

→ Transported from the adipose tissue to the muscle cell

→ Taken up into the muscle cell, which requires transporter molecules

→ "Activated" in a series of reactions that prepare the fatty acid molecule for the chemical reactions that will eventually produce energy from it

→ Oxidized (burned) to produce energy

Endurance training enhances every single one of the above steps, and it does so by stimulating the production of enzymes. These enzymes are like the workers on a production line, and their job is to catalyze and stimulate each of the above steps. More enzymes means greater productivity, allowing more fat to be used. Training also increases the number of mitochondria in the cell. Mitochondria are called the powerhouses of the cell; these tiny structures are where the chemical reactions that produce ATP take place when you are relying on oxygen use for energy production, as you are during endurance running. If you can increase the number of mitochondria, the analogy is that you are basically building new factories with new workers who are able to produce far more energy from fat.

The other big training-induced adaptation greatly reduces the stress of running. Recall what you felt like when you began running—to run even one mile represented an enormous stress on the body. This stress, as we saw in the Introduction with the story of Hans Selye's General Adaptation Principle, induces a whole range of responses called the sympathetic nervous system response, designed to help us survive. One of these responses is the stimulation of energy production from carbohydrate to meet our suddenly increased energy needs. However, with training, the relative magnitude of the stress is reduced, so instead of relying on rapid energy from carbohydrates, we can instead use fats, which are a little less accessible and hence not suitable for immediate energy production. A trained runner has a reduced sympathetic response and therefore a greater reliance on fat as a source of fuel.

As a result, a highly trained endurance runner is a fat-burning machine and can thus use far less carbohydrate than an untrained runner at the same running speed. This adaptation requires time, of course, since training effects do not occur overnight. It also requires a great deal of effort, so it's perhaps not surprising that people have looked at other, easier strategies in attempting to develop the same overall response of reduced carbohydrate use. The first of these is "fat-loading," or the use of a high-fat diet before an event.

Fat-Loading Diets: High-Fat Feeding to Stimulate Fat Burning

You may well be thinking that the last thing the world needs is yet another excuse to follow a high-fat diet. It seems that the default diet of the 21st century is a high-fat diet. However, the use of high-fat diets in athletes is regarded as one of the more interesting avenues of recent sports science research. The principle, which you are by now familiar with, is that if you can teach the body to use fat by feeding it with fat, then you rely less on carbohydrates and thus improve performance.

But why would high-fat diets increase the use of fat? Well, the body is a remarkable machine—it is able to adapt to the environment in numerous complex ways. And one of the ways it can adapt to the environment is by actually "learning" how to use the energy sources it is provided with. So, someone who eats a great deal of fat in his daily diet produces enzymes and transporters that help him use those fats more effectively, just as we saw in the previous section on training. The five steps that are required for fatty acid use are stimulated by fat feeding, though perhaps not quite to the extent that they're stimulated by training.

But does it work? The scientific research on high-fat diets and fat-loading is still equivocal.

Early evidence was promising and found that fat-loading actually improved performance during endurance exercise. More recently, however, that finding has not been repeated, and the difference between the studies is again in the nature of exercise being performed. It seems that time to fatigue and sub-maximal exercise may be improved, whereas time-trial performances with mixed intensity (which more closely simulate real racing) are not.

In terms of the protocol for high-fat diets, one thing must be remembered: If you start a long run with low glycogen levels, performance will be impaired. An undesired side effect of a high-fat diet is low carbohydrate intake and thus low glycogen levels. So when trying to fat-load, it's important that you allow one day of high carbohydrate intake immediately preceding the event, to top off glycogen levels. A typical protocol might, for example, consist of six days of high-fat diet followed by a single day of high-carbohydrate feeding to top off the glycogen tanks.

Our most important caution, however, is that there are very large differences in the individual responses to fat-loading and exercise. Some people perform slightly better on a high-fat diet, while others experience completely disastrous results. This large interindividual response is one of the most intriguing aspects of this area of research because it's not clear why some athletes thrive and others suffer on a high-fat diet. There is, however, evidence that some people are born "fat burners," while others are born "carbohydrate burners."

This evidence was provided by Dr. Julia Goedecke, an exercise physiologist at the University of Cape Town, who found that in any group of athletes, there is a roughly "normal" distribution of fuel use; some use far more fat and others use far more carbohydrate. While some of you are on the extremes of that curve and are excellent fat burners or carbohydrate burners, the vast majority of us exist in the middle of the range. It's possible to measure fuel use at rest and during exercise, and Goedecke's research has found that people who use more fat at rest are also more likely to use more fat during exercise. What it is that allows these people to do so is not yet known and is the subject of ongoing research. However, it is conceivable that some people, the fat burners, might thrive on a high-fat diet, while the carbohydrate burners are unable to meet their energy needs during exercise unless they have abundant carbohydrate stores.

Given our lack of understanding of the interindividual responses to high levels of fat intake, the prudent approach, for now, is to focus on a high-carbohydrate diet and make sure that you are not compromising performance by depleting your glycogen stores before exercise. In the future, it may well be possible to screen runners in order to establish whether they are adapted for fat or carbohydrate use and then to prescribe targeted nutritional strategies to improve their performance. But for the average runner engaging in marathons and shorter races, adapting to a high-fat diet is unlikely to yield significant benefits. This is because even during a marathon, it is easy enough to ingest enough carbohydrate during the race to help the liver stave off the "bonk." But if you have graduated to ultraendurance events such as the Western States 100, experimenting with a high-fat diet might be a sensible step to take.

Until fuel-type screening arrives, though, a high-carbohydrate diet during training is perhaps the most crucial thing for runners to get right, and even carbo-loading is less significant than the training diet. Once you're in the race, of course, the regular ingestion of carbohydrates is critical. Training is the nonnegotiable variable that will improve performance, including the increased capacity to use fat as a fuel.

Fat-Burning Zones and the Use of Energy Stores during Running

Now that we've looked at the four sources of energy during running and how your diet and training will help you maximize your fuel economy, which source of energy your body will rely on most at different times and how this should influence your performance and training remain to be discussed.

The relative use of different fuels during exercise is an area that has been open to a couple of myths and "urban legends" in the past, and it warrants a logical discussion in order to tease out the scientific fact from the marketing fiction. The two myths are:

1. To burn more fat, it's best to train at low intensity, in the "fat-burning zone."

2. The body "switches" to fat-burning during a run.

Let's tackle these myths one at a time.

1. THE EFFECT OF EXERCISE INTENSITY ON FUEL USE: DOES THE "FAT-BURNING ZONE" EXIST?

The first myth concerns the concept that there is a zone or an exercise intensity at which you must run in order to burn fat. Why is this important? Because it says that if you run too fast, you'll stop burning fat and instead use only carbohydrates; therefore, low-intensity training is best for both weight loss (since by "weight loss" we really mean "fat loss") and teaching your body how to use fat for muscle work.

What does science say about this notion? The graph on page 146 comes from a study done back in 1993 by Hans Romijn, a Dutch researcher who was able to measure how much of an exercising athlete's total energy was coming from fat as opposed to carbohydrates at a range of different exercise intensities. Remember, the prevalent theory is that you burn more fat at lower exercise intensities, or slower running speeds.

At first glance, Romijn's results seem to bear this notion. Look, for example, at the bars on the far left, which are measured at

25 percent of VO₂ max. This is very low exercise intensity, comparable to a moderately paced walk for most runners. What Romijn found is that at this intensity, approximately 85 percent of the total energy comes from fat stores, either in the muscle or from the adipose tissue, and only 15 percent comes from glycogen. As we move up to the higher exercise intensities, the relative contribution of fat goes down. By the time we hit 85 percent of VO₂ max (roughly the intensity at which

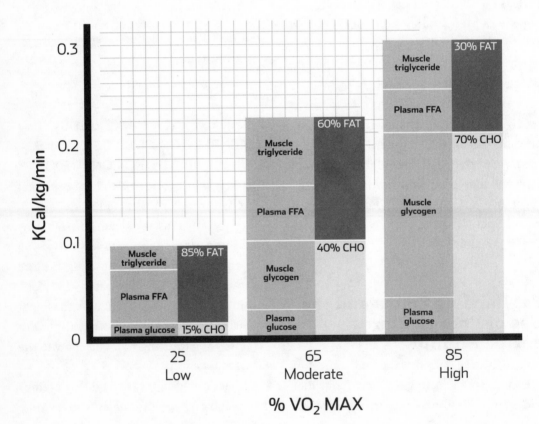

you'd run a 10-K race), only a third of the energy comes from fat, and muscle glycogen provides the bulk of the required energy.

So, the problem is solved—low intensity is best. Or is it? Consider the following offer:

If we said that you had a choice between taking 50 percent of the money in Ross's wallet or 20 percent of the money in Jonathan's wallet (Matt is broke and has no money in his wallet right now.), you'd want to know how much money there was in each wallet before making your decision. Why? Because you recognize that it's not important to have a greater percentage, but rather a greater *total* amount of money. Ross's wallet (which is usually empty) would be a bad choice, since you'd be getting 50 percent of very little. On the other hand, if you chose Jonathan's wallet, you might be getting only 20 percent, but it would be a great deal more in total than your other option.

The same goes for fat-burning. If your goal is to lose weight or teach your body to burn fat, then your primary objective should be to burn the greatest total amount of fat during training. Look again at the graph showing Romijn's research. At 25 percent, most of the energy comes from fat, but the total is very small. If you move to 65 percent, then you get less energy from fat (only 60 percent of the total, compared with 85 percent at slow speeds), but the key is that you would burn almost two and a half times the *total* energy

(as shown on the y-axis). Therefore, at 65 percent VO$_2$ max, you actually end up burning about 50 percent more fat than at slow speeds.

The myth that lower exercise intensity is better for fat-burning is therefore incorrect; if you want to maximize the total amount of fat you burn, then exercising at a moderate intensity is best. It does get a little more complicated than this because if you keep exercising harder, then eventually you do reach a point at which fat use actually goes down. This happens because the body shuts down circulation to the fat cells, so the energy becomes "trapped" there and can't be used. The true answer to our question is that you should aim for a moderate intensity—too slow doesn't help, and very fast becomes restrictive, but you get optimal results in the middle. There is no fat-burning zone, just a commonsense approach to making the most of fat use during exercise.

It's worth noting that even though you are burning fat at 65 percent of VO$_2$ max, the total amount of fat you burn is less than 1 gram per minute. Therefore, even if you exercise for an hour at this intensity, you will burn less than 60 grams of fat. A normal body fat percentage equates to 10,000 to 15,000 grams of fat in the body, so you can see that burning even 1 gram of fat per minute is hardly going to dent this stockpile. Instead, if weight loss is your aim, focus on creating an energy deficit (burning more calories than you eat each day). If you are running 30 to 60 minutes per workout, then this is easily accomplished, and if you maintain this deficit, you will indeed lose some fat and improve your body composition.

In other words, if your primary goal is weight loss, think in terms of the total number of calories you burn through exercise, not the types of calories (whether carbs or fat). The types of calories you burn during exercise are irrelevant to weight loss because of a phenomenon called *energy partitioning*. It works like this: After you complete a low-intensity workout in which you burn mostly fat, your glycogen stores remain fairly full, so few of the calories you eat during the rest of the day will be used to replenish your muscles' glycogen stores. Some calories might be used to create new fat stores. But after you finish a high-intensity workout in which you burn a lot of carbohydrate, your glycogen stores are greatly depleted, and many of the calories you consume later in the day will be used to replenish these stores; few or none will be stored as body fat. And, in fact, your body is likely to break down some stored body

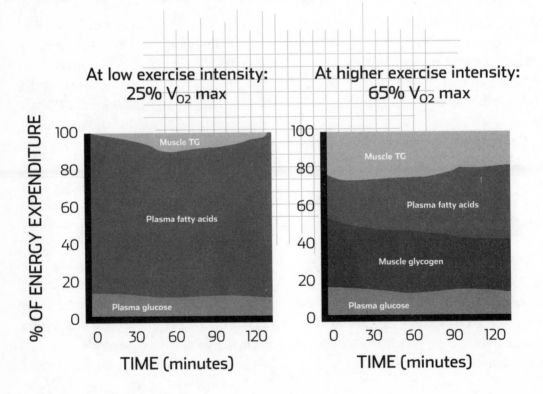

At low exercise intensity: 25% V_{O2} max

At higher exercise intensity: 65% V_{O2} max

% OF ENERGY EXPENDITURE

Muscle TG

Plasma fatty acids

Plasma glucose

Muscle TG

Plasma fatty acids

Muscle glycogen

Plasma glucose

TIME (minutes)

TIME (minutes)

Fuel Use

Breakdown of typical foods containing 50 grams of carbohydrates and the amount of each food required for a high-carbohydrate meal

Foods with 50 grams of carbohydrates	For 80 kilograms, you'd need . . .
3 slices of bread	48 slices
3 medium-size muffins	48 muffins
1 cup baked beans	16 cups
3 medium potatoes	48 potatoes
1.5 cups of rice	24 cups
500 ml of cola	8 liters of cola
250 ml of yogurt	4 liters of yogurt

fat to supply postexercise energy needs, because the high-priority glycogen restoration would be slowed down if your body drew on carbs for these needs.

You can see that when you consider the workout and postworkout period combined, everything balances out in terms of fat and carbohydrate use and replenishment. Ultimately, all that matters with respect to weight loss is the total number of calories burned during exercise. If you generally eat enough carbohydrate to replenish your glycogen stores and enough protein to maintain your muscles, then your body has to break down fat to make up the difference between the number of calories you burn daily and the number of calories you eat, regardless of your preferred running intensity.

2. A FAT-BURNING "SWITCH": DO WE SUDDENLY SWITCH TO FAT AS FUEL DURING EXERCISE?

The second myth concerns the perception that during running, we use carbohydrates up to a point and then suddenly "switch" to fats. In other words, it holds that there is a distinct moment at which fat use changes. This notion has implications for your training because if you wish to burn fat, then you would have to exercise beyond this switching point in order to do so.

For the answer, we refer to Romijn's study (opposite). The graph shows the contributions (as a percentage of total) of the four energy stores to total energy production during two hours of exercise at two different intensities: 25 percent of VO_2 max (moderate walking

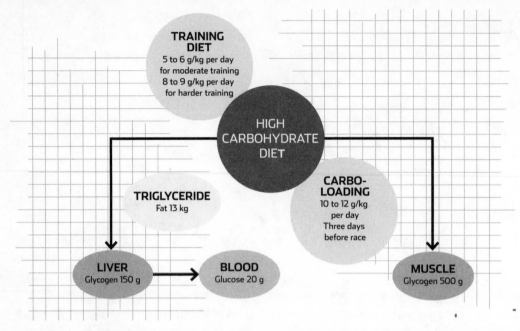

Figure showing the physiological role of high-carbohydrate diets on energy stores during running, including summarized guidelines for optimal carbohydrate intake

speed) and 65 percent of VO$_2$ max (your pace on a long, steady run).

It shows the following:

→ There is definitely no switch point at which fat suddenly becomes the main source of energy. At both intensities, there are gradual changes in the contributions from fats and carbohydrates, but at no point does the use of carbohydrates drop off to be replaced by fat.

→ The general pattern, particularly at the moderate exercise intensity, is that over time, you use fewer carbohydrates, while the contribution from fats increases progressively. At the start, the ratio is roughly 50:50, whereas after two hours, fats make up 60 percent of the total energy.

→ Both fats and carbohydrates are used from the very first minute, and the main change is that, over time, the contribution from the intramuscular stores goes down, replaced by circulating energy (fatty acids from adipose tissue and glucose from the liver).

The implication of these findings is that you do not need to exercise for 2 hours before your body starts using fat. Of course, there are many reasons for a marathon runner to do long runs, and improving fat use is one of them. But it's not a case where you gain little benefit for the first 90 minutes and then suddenly start to use fats. Instead, you use all four sources from the outset, and the relative contribution changes gradually over time.

For both weight loss and performance, therefore, it's more important to get the intensity and duration right in order to optimize total fat use.

Conclusion

In this section, we've looked at how the body uses fuels to make energy during running.

We've seen how the interaction between training and diet is able to alter the use of the different fuel stores, eventually resulting in improved performance. Training adaptations, which increase the body's capacity to use fat as a fuel, are perhaps the most crucial and are moderated by various diet strategies, such as carbo-loading, fat-loading, and ingestion of carbohydrates on the run.

These are very broad and general dietary strategies, however. In order to further understand the role of diet in performance, we must look in more detail at what you should eat as a runner. And this is where we head next.

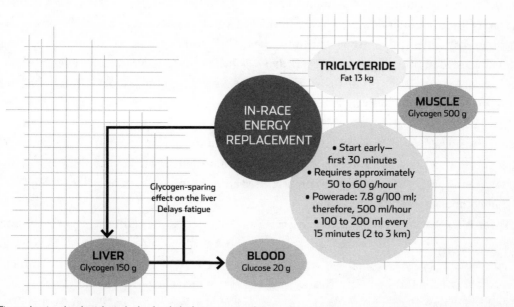

Figure showing the physiological role of carbohydrate ingestion *during* exercise on energy stores, including summarized guidelines for optimal carbohydrate intake

[Chapter 9]

All You Can Eat

One-third of the calories in the average American diet come from processed foods with high caloric density and low nutrient value (candy, processed baked goods, fast food, and so forth). The average runner doesn't eat much better. Even many elite runners are careless in their dietary habits. In an interview on the New York Road Runners Web site, two-time Olympic steeplechaser Anthony Famiglietti described his diet as "all junk." A segment about Fam's eating habits included in his self-produced DVD *Run Like Hell* is entitled "Worst Diet Ever." Record-breaking miler Alan Webb is said to live on cheese steaks and Chinese takeout. The food choices of these great runners appear to lend credence to the notion, held by many everyday runners, that it really doesn't matter what they eat. Their heavy exercise habit allows them to "get away with" eating whatever they want. It is certainly true that runners in heavy training can often eat whatever they want and as much as they want without getting fat. But can they do so without sacrificing performance, through compromised antioxidant defenses, less-elastic blood vessels, and other factors?

The truth is that we just don't know. We certainly can't accept the eating habits of Webb and Famiglietti as scientific proof that "anything goes" in the diet of a runner in heavy training, because nobody has yet studied the performance effects of an improved diet in elite runners whose habitual diets are poor. In any case, world-class runners who burn 2,000 to 3,000 calories a day through training alone must consume so much food to keep from wasting away that they might take in enough vitamins, minerals, and antioxidants to support optimal performance despite the low nutrient density of their food choices. If so—and it may or may not be so—then that's great for them, but it certainly doesn't give license to everyday runners, who may burn only 500 to 1,000 calories a day in training, to emulate their sporting heroes' gustatory habits with impunity.

We believe that the more science learns about how foods affect endurance athletic performance and recovery, the more benefits we will see in consuming wholesome foods, and the more liabilities of consuming unhealthy foods. But we might have to wait a while for this research to be done. Sports nutrition research is dominated by short-term studies on nutritional supplements such as creatine and amino acids. There are surprisingly few good studies on the effects of real food. That's too bad, because real food has a much bigger impact on athletic performance than supplements, which, by definition, can do no more than *supplement* the benefits of eating the right foods. And most supplements don't even do that much, as the research clearly proves. They're useless.

The reason so few real food studies are performed in exercise science is that they are more difficult to execute and fund. It's far easier to obtain funding from a nutritional supplement company that stands to profit from a study demonstrating benefits associated with taking a particular supplement that the company sells. Summaries of these studies in turn dominate the sports nutrition content of the information channels that communicate nutrition information to athletes, such as running magazines, whose pages are filled with advertisements for the companies that funded the studies in the first place. This unfortunate reality leads to a skewed sense that sports nutrition is all about choosing and using the right supplements, when it's really all about choosing the best foods. You can find no better evidence of this than the fact that most of the world's best runners come from Kenya and Ethiopia, where nutritional supplementation is not widely practiced.

Do runners then have no solid science to use to guide their eating choices? Thankfully, there's particularly good information about the effects of different ratios of macronutrients (carbohydrate, fat, and protein) on exercise performance, which we discussed in the previous chapter. Due to our society's intense interest in managing body weight, we also know a lot about what runners can do to optimize their body weight for performance—and that's the topic of the next chapter. Finally, it's important to bear in mind that there is a very high degree of overlap between endurance fitness and basic health. Science has accumulated a wealth of information about how humans should eat for basic health. In taking advantage of this information, runners will surely enhance their running performance in myriad ways, even if we still have a lot to learn about the details.

Eating for health and, by extension, for performance is the subject of this chapter.

Eating for Health and Performance

In many ways, general health and running fitness are nearly the same. For example, a lean body composition (low body fat percentage) not only reduces the risk of chronic diseases such as heart disease and diabetes but also aids athletic performance by reducing the energy cost of movement. A strong antioxidant defense system is another key characteristic of health and running performance. The antioxidant defense system (which we'll learn more about in Chapter 14) is a complex network of enzymes and other chemical compounds, including dietary nutrients, that protect cells against the sorts of chemical damage that cause muscle fatigue during running, postexercise muscle soreness after running, aging over the long term—and even diseases such as cancer. Diet affects body composition, the antioxidant defense system, and every other characteristic of health and physical fitness. In general, the same healthy diet that maximizes overall health will most likely also maximize running performance.

Scientists determine what constitutes a healthy diet by studying how specific foods and dietary patterns affect disease risk, body functioning, and mortality and longevity. This research has not led the scientific community to any consensus on the definition of a healthy diet. There are strong disagreements over a variety of specific issues, such as whether healthy individuals should minimize salt intake to reduce the risk of high blood pressure. (It seems that some individuals are more sensitive to salt than others and probably should. But everyone should consume salt in moderation, to be on the safe side.) But most such controversies are on the periphery of the effort to define a healthy diet. Almost all nutrition scientists agree on the biggest issues. We summarize this near consensus about diet, organized by basic food types, in the following set of recommendations.

FRUITS AND VEGETABLES

Fresh fruits and vegetables should account for a majority of daily food portions (three or more servings of each). Those who eat the most vegetables have lower risks of many chronic diseases and also live longer. The mechanisms underlying these benefits—such as strengthened antioxidant defenses—may also directly benefit running performance. For example, in one study, the addition of cherry juice (which is rich in antioxidants called anthocyanins) to the diet of competitive rowers significantly reduced the amount of strength loss and muscle soreness they experienced after a strength test designed to cause muscle damage, compared with a group of fellow rowers who received a placebo.

GRAINS

Grains are not necessary for general health, and indeed they were not a significant part of the human diet until relatively recently in history. Nevertheless, a diet containing a fair amount of grains (up to six servings daily) can be perfectly healthy. And because grains are the richest sources of carbohydrate, and runners need plenty of carbohydrate, runners really have no cause to limit their grain consumption.

Most or all of the grains you consume should be whole grains such as brown rice, which offer more fiber, vitamins, and minerals than refined grains such as white rice. Studies have shown that individuals who consume the greatest amounts of whole grains are less likely to be overweight than those who eat fewer whole grains. This is true in part because whole grains provide more fullness per calorie, so those who eat a lot of them eat less. Whole grains also typically release energy into the bloodstream more slowly and provide a host of other health benefits, including improved function of the digestive system, reducing the risk of colon cancer and other diseases.

For example, a study from Pennsylvania State University found that a diet rich in whole grains may promote weight loss and reduce the risk of chronic diseases such as diabetes. Participants in the study were 25 men and 25 women with metabolic syndrome (a cluster of characteristics consisting of abdominal obesity, high LDL cholesterol and low HDL cholesterol, high blood pressure, insulin resistance or glucose intolerance, and systemic inflammation). All 50 subjects were placed on the same weight-loss diet for 12 weeks, except that half of them were counseled to consume all of their grains in the form of whole grains. Members of both groups lost weight—8 to 11 pounds—but those in the whole grain group lost more abdominal fat. In addition, the whole grain group exhibited a 38 percent decrease in C-reactive protein, a marker of whole-body inflammation, which underlies various chronic diseases.

Whole grain foods are particularly good choices for preworkout meals. That's because they top off the body's glycogen stores without causing the blood sugar crash that may result from eating a meal of refined grains without much fat or protein.

BEANS, NUTS, AND SEEDS

Nuts and seeds are among the best plant sources of fats and proteins and should have a regular place in the diet (three or more servings per week). Certain types of beans, nuts, and seeds—particularly soybeans, walnuts, and flaxseeds—also provide essential omega-3 polyunsaturated fats that are often deficient in the typical diet. Omega-3 fats support nervous system and cardiovascular function. Their health benefits are well known, but their benefits for athletes are just beginning to emerge in the scientific literature. We'll explain momentarily.

MEAT AND FISH

Meat and fish are not necessary for optimal health but are quite healthful in moderation (one to two servings a day). They are excellent sources of protein and micronutrients such as iron and vitamin B_{12}. Wild fish and organic meats are often leaner and more nutritious and should be chosen whenever possible.

Some meats are better than others. The leaner they are—that is, the less fat they contain—the better. As a general rule, try to avoid meats that contain more than 10 percent fat. You can find lean pieces of turkey and chicken and lean cuts of beef, pork, and lamb that are below this limit. Most of the fat in meats is saturated fat, and most Americans eat too much saturated fat and not enough unsaturated fat. The ratio of unsaturated to saturated fats in the typical American diet is roughly 1:2. The ideal ratio is just the reverse, 2:1 (that is, twice as many unsaturated fats as saturated fats), since saturated fats tend to increase LDL cholesterol levels. That said, not all unsaturated fats are good, either—the trans fats (which are formed from partial hydrogenation and are found in commercial fats and hard-block margarines) also increase LDL cholesterol and decrease HDL cholesterol, both of which are undesirable changes.

If you eat only one type of animal food, make it cold-water fish such as wild salmon, anchovies, mackerel, herring, and sardines. These fish contain large amounts of DHA and EPA, the two main omega-3 fats found in animals. Try to eat such fish at least two times a week. Also consider taking a fish oil supplement every day if you are not getting this amount of fish in your diet or if you have cardiovascular disease. Research has shown that the oils from the above fish provide significant health benefits and possibly some exercise performance benefits, too. For example, fish oils increase the elasticity of the blood vessels, which not only reduces heart disease risk but also may enhance cardiac efficiency during exercise. In one study, fish oil supplementation reduced the heart rate at a fixed running intensity in elite rugby players.

Generally we are not big fans of supplements, but in the case of omega-3 fats, we make an exception. Omega-3s are very difficult to obtain in adequate amounts through the diet if you don't eat two servings of fish per week. In a recent position statement based on a comprehensive review of the relevant literature, the American Dietetic Association determined that omega-3 acids from fish oil supplements appear to be as bioavailable and bioactive as those in whole fish.

DAIRY FOODS

Dairy foods are also not necessary for optimal health but are healthful in moderation (up to three servings per day). If you do include dairy foods in your diet, consider consuming reduced-fat versions of such foods instead of the regular, full-fat versions, which are high in saturated fat. While there's nothing inherently unhealthy about saturated fat, there's simply way too much of it—especially in relation to the amount of unsaturated fat consumed—in the typical diet, so it's a good idea to cut it out where you can.

Due to their richness in high-quality proteins and carbohydrates, low-fat dairy foods are an excellent source of postworkout nutrition for muscle recovery. A recent English study found that individuals exhibited less muscle damage and recovered their muscle strength faster when they consumed milk after a workout then when they consumed either a sports drink or water.

SWEETS

Sugar accounts for 17 percent of calories in the average American's diet. That's far too much. Increases in sugar consumption are largely responsible for the rise in overweight and obesity that has occurred over the past 30 years. Avoid foods and beverages with added sugar as much as your willpower allows.

FRIED FOODS

Frying adds a lot of calories to foods. Weight control is much more difficult on a diet that includes a lot of fried foods. Many fried foods also contain artery-clogging trans fats. As with sweets, limit your consumption of fried foods to the occasional treat.

Keeping Score

If you're like most runners, your diet is probably not as high in quality as it could be. An effective way to improve your diet quality is to grade, or score, the quality of your current diet and continue to score your diet quality as you make efforts to improve it. Nutrition scientists have come up with various ways of measuring diet quality. They are a bit too complex to be useful to the average runner, so we've created our own simplified diet quality scoring system, which you will find very easy to work with. Although it is rather too simple for scientific use, its scientific underpinnings are solid enough to make a significant difference in how well you nourish your body for health and running performance.

Here's how to use it: Each time you eat or drink something, look it up in the Diet Quality Score (DQS) table (page 158) and note the point score associated with it. If it's your first serving of that particular type of food or drink that day, use the score in the "1st" column. If it's your second serving of that type of food or drink, then use the score in the "2nd" column, and so forth. Start with breakfast and keep a running tally throughout the day. After following your last meal, snack, or drink before bedtime, note your total DQS for the day. Tomorrow, start over.

As you'll see, there are 11 different types of foods listed on the DQS table. They closely match but do not precisely match the categories presented in the previous section. Those shaded green are high-quality foods and drinks that add positive points to your DQS score, unless you eat too much of them. Those shaded red are low-quality foods that subtract points from your DQS.

Perhaps the most striking aspect of the table on first glance is the fact that many foods and drinks are scored differently depending on how many times you've already consumed them on a given day. For example, your first, second, and third daily servings of low-fat dairy add 1 point each to your DQS score, but your fourth serving adds none, your

fifth serving subtracts 1, and your sixth serving subtracts 2. How come?

The reason is that consuming one serving of low-fat dairy per day will tend to make you leaner and healthier than consuming none, but two servings are better still, and three servings are best of all, while adding a fourth serving will bring no additional benefits; after five servings, low-fat dairy becomes too much of a good thing. The same rationale applies to all the food and drink types that score differently depending on how many servings of that kind of food or drink you've already consumed.

Diet Quality Score (DQS)

	1st	2nd	3rd	4th	5th	6th
Fruit	2	2	2	1	0	0
Vegetable	2	2	2	1	0	0
Lean protein	2	2	1	0	0	-1
Whole grain	2	2	1	0	0	-1
Low-fat dairy	1	1	1	0	-1	-2
Omega-3 fats	2	0	0	0	-1	-1
Refined grain	-1	-1	-2	-2	-2	-2
Sweet	-2	-2	-2	-2	-2	-2
Fried food	-2	-2	-2	-2	-2	-2
Full-fat dairy	-1	-1	-2	-2	-2	-2
Fatty protein	-1	-1	-2	-2	-2	-2

A lean protein is any type of fish or meat that's less than 10 percent fat, as well as nuts and soy foods. Count your first serving of low-

fat dairy each day as a lean protein, too—because it is. A fatty protein is any meat that contains more than 10 percent fat. Foods that count as omega-3 servings include salmon, halibut, snapper, shrimp, scallops, mackerel, anchovies, flaxseeds, walnuts, and soy foods. Any foods and beverages containing more than 10 grams of added sugar count as sweets. Foods that cover two categories should be scored twice. For example, count salmon as both a lean protein and an omega-3 fat; count ice cream as a sweet and a full-fat dairy food. The exception is low-fat dairy foods—only the first daily serving should also be counted as a lean protein, as mentioned above.

In order to use the DQS effectively, you need to know how to count servings of the various food types listed on the DQS table. The following table has enough information to guide you through the process of determining your DQS for a day's eating. The amounts don't have to be exact. Use your common sense. A dab of ketchup on a hot dog does not count as a vegetable serving. A very large serving of steak should count as two servings of lean or fatty protein, depending on the cut. Note that the table contains guidelines for high-quality foods only. Any amount of an unhealthy food (within reason—you don't have to count a single sip of soda or two french fries) counts as a serving.

The maximum DQS you can achieve in one day—by consuming four fruits, four vegetables, three lean proteins, three whole grains, three servings of low-fat dairy, three servings of omega-3 fats, and zero sweets, fried foods, full-fat dairy servings, or fatty proteins—is 32 points. Very few people consistently eat this well. You certainly don't have to accumulate 32 DQS points day after day to maximize your health and running performance. But you probably will have to improve your diet quality to some degree. How much depends on your current DQS and on factors such as your age, genetic factors that influence your metabolism, and so forth.

If your current DQS is far below 32 points, don't feel obligated to radically transform your diet in a single day. Habits are hard to break. All too often, when people try to change their dietary habits too much too soon, they experience a motivational burnout and return to their old ways. Therefore, unless you're confident that you can make your "perfect" new diet stick, we recommend that you

Fruit	1 whole apple, banana, pear, orange, etc. 1 handful of berries, grapes, etc. 8 oz 100% fruit juice
Vegetable	½ cup cooked spinach, beans, etc. 1 cup salad Fist-size portion broccoli, carrots, etc.
Lean protein	Open-hand-size portion meat, fish 1 egg or 2 egg whites Handful nuts
Whole grain	1–2 slices whole grain bread 1 cup whole grain breakfast cereal, whole grain pasta Fist-size portion brown rice, barley, etc.
Low-Fat dairy	8 oz skim milk 2 slices low-fat cheese 8 oz low-fat yogurt
Omega-3 fats	Open-hand-size portion wild salmon ¼ cup ground flaxseeds ¼ cup almonds 1 serving fish oil

alter current habits gradually. Don't change them any more than is necessary to get the results you desire. Note the DQS that's associated with these new patterns and use that as your standard going forward.

A good way to begin improving your diet is to substitute some of the unhealthy foods you are currently eating with healthier alternatives. There are several very simple types of substitutions that almost suggest themselves:

Instead of this:	Eat (or drink) this:
Refined-grain food (e.g., white rice)	Whole-grain food (e.g., brown rice)
Fatty protein (e.g., 80% lean ground beef)	Lean protein (e.g., 95% lean ground beef)
Full-fat dairy (e.g., ice cream)	Low-fat dairy (e.g., fat-free yogurt)
Sweet (e.g., ice cream)	Fruit (e.g., mixed berries)
Fried food (e.g., fried chicken)	Non-fried alternative (e.g., grilled skinless chicken breast)
Caloric beverage (e.g., Red Bull)	Water

In addition to making the substitutions suggested in the table above, adding more fruit and vegetable servings to your diet (assuming you eat fewer than four servings of each daily) is a very effective way to increase your DQS score. Fruits are great as snacks and desserts. One daily serving of 100 percent fruit juice counts as a fruit serving as well. Adding a salad to your lunch or dinner is a great way to increase your vegetable consumption. A large, meal-size salad counts as two servings of vegetables. Naturally, you'll need to "make room" for these additional vegetables by eating less of, or replacing, other things. For example, if you normally eat a whole sandwich at lunch, eat a salad and half a sandwich instead.

If your current DQS is below zero, you might be tempted to raise it by simply eliminating unhealthy food servings from your diet. After all, zero points is better than negative points, right? Not really. You'll raise your DQS much more by replacing unhealthy foods with healthy alternatives. This greater "point swing" reflects the fact that eating something healthy is almost always better than eating nothing. Replacing unhealthy foods is also better than eliminating them, because it does not increase your hunger level.

Here's an example of how this process works. Martha is a runner who currently has a very poor diet. She will improve her diet quality with a gradual approach in which she focuses on just one meal per week. Even so, as you will see, Martha's overall diet quality will drastically improve after just six weeks. To keep things simple, we will make step-by-step modifications to a single typical day's menu for Martha.

Day 0

Before she begins Positive Eating, Martha's diet is fairly typical—and pretty bad. Her DQS is pushed deep into the negative (-12, to be exact) by a mixture of sweetened beverages and other sugary treats, fried foods, whole-milk dairy foods, and refined grains.

Meal	Diet contents	DQS category
Breakfast	Bagel with cream cheese 16 oz caffe latte	1 refined grain 1 full-fat dairy 1 sweet
Lunch	Ham and cheese sandwich Bag of potato chips 12 oz can of soda Apple	1 refined grain 1 fatty protein 1 full-fat dairy 1 fried food 1 sweet 1 fruit
Dinner	Spaghetti with meat sauce Green salad Garlic bread Wine	1 refined grain 1 fatty protein 2 vegetables
Snack	Bowl of ice cream	1 sweet 1 full-fat dairy
Total DQS Points		**-12**

Week 1

Martha begins her diet overhaul by replacing her low-quality breakfast with a high-quality one. She also adds a serving of fish oil to her daily nutrition regimen. These changes increase her DQS by 10 points.

Meal	Diet contents	DQS category
Breakfast	Old-fashioned oatmeal with raisins + fat-free milk Coffee Fish oil	1 whole grain 1 fruit 1 low-fat dairy/lean protein 1 omega-3 fat
Lunch	Ham and cheese sandwich Bag of potato chips 12 oz can of soda Apple	1 refined grain 1 fatty protein 1 full-fat dairy 1 fried food 1 sweet 1 fruit
Dinner	Spaghetti with meat sauce Green salad Garlic bread Wine	1 refined grain 1 fatty protein 2 vegetables
Snack	Bowl of ice cream	1 sweet 1 full-fat dairy
Total DQS Points		**-2**

Week 2

In Week 2, Martha adds a healthy midmorning snack to her eating schedule. Her DQS is no longer negative!

Meal	Diet contents	DQS category
Breakfast	Old-fashioned oatmeal with raisins + fat-free milk Coffee Fish oil	1 whole grain 1 fruit 1 low-fat dairy/lean protein 1 omega-3 fat
Midmorning snack	Raw veggies dipped in low-fat ranch dressing	1 vegetable
Lunch	Ham and cheese sandwich Bag of potato chips 12 oz can of soda Apple	1 refined grain 1 fatty protein 1 full-fat dairy 1 fried food 1 sweet 1 fruit
Dinner	Spaghetti with meat sauce Green salad Garlic bread Wine	1 refined grain 1 fatty protein 2 vegetables 1 sweet
Snack	Bowl of ice cream	1 sweet 1 full-fat dairy
Total DQS Points		**0**

Week 3

Martha's lunch comes up for transformation in Week 3. By replacing her sandwich with a chicken Caesar salad wrap and her soda with water, she boosts her DQS by another 11 points. As you see, Martha chooses to allow herself to keep the small indulgence of a bag of potato chips for now. That's okay.

Meal time	Diet contents	DQS category
Breakfast	Old-fashioned oatmeal with raisins + fat-free milk Coffee Fish oil	1 whole grain 1 fruit 1 low-fat dairy/lean protein 1 omega-3 fat
Midmorning snack	Raw veggies dipped in low-fat ranch dressing	1 vegetable
Lunch	Chicken Caesar salad wrap (whole wheat) Bag of potato chips Water Apple	1 whole grain 1 lean protein 1 vegetable 1 fried food 1 fruit
Dinner	Spaghetti with meat sauce Green salad Garlic bread Wine	1 refined grain 1 fatty protein 2 vegetables 1 sweet
Snack	Bowl of ice cream	1 sweet 1 full-fat dairy
Total DQS Points		**+11**

Week 4

The only change for Martha in Week 4 is the addition of a healthy midafternoon snack.

Isn't it great that you can increase your diet quality by eating *more* food?

Meal	Diet contents	DQS category
Breakfast	Old-fashioned oatmeal with raisins + fat-free milk Coffee Fish oil	1 whole-grain 1 fruit 1 low-fat dairy/lean protein 1 omega-3 fat
Midmorning snack	Raw veggies dipped in low-fat ranch dressing	1 vegetables
Lunch	Chicken Caesar salad wrap (whole wheat) Bag of potato chips Water Apple	1 whole grain 1 lean protein 1 vegetable 1 fried food 1 fruit
Midafternoon snack	Trail mix (dried fruit and nuts)	½ lean protein ½ fruit
Dinner	Spaghetti with meat sauce Green salad Garlic bread Wine	1 refined grain 1 fatty protein 2 vegetables 1 sweet
Evening snack	Bowl of ice cream	1 sweet 1 full-fat dairy
Total DQS Points		**+13**

Week 5

Martha's original dinner wasn't too bad, but by switching to a lean protein and replacing a refined grain with a whole grain, she nets 15

DQS points. She decides to keep her relaxing evening glass of wine.

Meal time	Diet contents	DQS category
Breakfast	Old-fashioned oatmeal with raisins + fat-free milk Coffee Fish oil	1 whole grain 1 fruit 1 low-fat dairy/lean protein 1 omega-3 fat
Midmorning snack	Raw veggies dipped in low-fat ranch dressing	1 vegetable
Lunch	Chicken Caesar salad wrap (whole wheat) Bag of potato chips Water Apple	1 whole grain 1 lean protein 1 vegetable 1 fried food 1 fruit
Midafternoon snack	Trail mix (dried fruit and nuts)	½ lean protein ½ fruit
Dinner	Broiled salmon Steamed green beans Brown rice Wine	1 whole grain 1 lean protein 1 vegetable
Evening snack	Bowl of ice cream	1 sweet 1 full-fat dairy
Total DQS Points		**+19**

Week 6

Martha completes her diet overhaul by replacing her evening bowl of ice cream (which counts as a sweet and a full-fat dairy food) with a healthier, fruit-based treat for her sweet tooth. Her DQS is now 24 points!

Meal	Diet contents	DQS category
Breakfast	Old-fashioned oatmeal with raisins + full-fat milk Coffee Fish oil	1 whole grain 1 fruit 1 low-fat dairy/lean protein 1 omega-3 fat
Midmorning snack	Raw veggies dipped in low-fat ranch dressing	1 vegetable
Lunch	Chicken Caesar salad wrap (whole wheat) Bag of potato chips Water Apple	1 whole grain 1 lean protein 1 vegetable 1 fried food 1 fruit
Midafternoon snack	Trail mix (dried fruit and nuts)	1 lean protein 1 vegetable
Dinner	Broiled salmon Steamed green beans Brown rice Wine	1 whole grain 1 lean protein 1 vegetable 1 sweet 1 healthy fat
Snack	Vanilla low-fat yogurt with banana slices	1 low-fat dairy 1 fruit
Total DQS Points		**+24**

What about Caffeine and Alcohol?

Surely you noticed that coffee and wine remain on Martha's overhauled diet, although caffeine and alcohol are not included as positives or negatives in the Diet Quality Score Table. So, are caffeine and alcohol good for you or bad for you?

Both are good in moderation (one to two cups of coffee, one to two glasses of wine per day). Caffeine seems to be most beneficial when consumed in those foods and beverages in which it occurs naturally: mainly coffee, tea, and dark chocolate. Moderate coffee consumption has a number of proven health benefits. The health benefits of coffee come from both its caffeine content and its unique blend of antioxidants. According to Harvard Medical School, "Studies show that the risk for type 2 diabetes is lower among regular coffee drinkers than among those who don't drink it. Also, coffee may reduce the risk of developing gallstones, discourage the development of colon cancer, improve cognitive function, reduce the risk of liver damage in people at high risk for liver disease, and reduce the risk of Parkinson's disease." Caffeine also enhances mood and, yes, even exercise performance.

Moderate alcohol consumption has been shown to improve heart health by increasing levels of HDL cholesterol and lowering levels of LDL cholesterol and also through other mechanisms. A recent study from the Medical University of South Carolina found that middle-aged women who began drinking one alcoholic beverage per day experienced a 38 percent reduction in cardiovascular disease risk after four years compared with women who remained nondrinkers.

In addition to boosting heart health, moderate alcohol consumption is proven to reduce the risk of type 2 diabetes by improving insulin sensitivity and reducing systemic inflammation. Moderate drinkers even tend to live longer than both heavy drinkers and teetotalers.

Wine is an especially good alcoholic beverage choice because it is rich in antioxidants. Red wine contains significantly higher levels of antioxidants than white wine.

What is the definition of "moderate drinking"? The greatest benefits seem to come from one to two drinks (one serving of wine is an eight-ounce glass) per day. Any more and the negative effects of alcohol on the liver, the brain, the waistline, and other body parts start to outweigh the positives. Also, it's important to clearly understand that it is not necessary to consume alcohol for optimal health. If you're currently a nondrinker for personal, family, health, or moral reasons, you shouldn't feel pressure to change.

[Chapter 10]

Leaner, Lighter, Faster

Runners come in all shapes and sizes. Even among the elite of the sport, there is a great deal of variety in physical proportions. For example, the fastest female marathon runner of all time, England's Paula Radcliffe, is tall at 5'8", while the fastest male marathon runner of all time, Ethiopia's Haile Gebrselassie, is short, at 5'3".

There are limits to the diversity of body types at the front of the pack, however. Nearly all world-class runners are skinny—meaning they have a low height-to-weight ratio, or body mass index—and lean—meaning they have a low body fat percentage. In fact, long-distance runners are among the leanest athletes in any sport. Exercise physiologists William McArdle of the City College of New York and Frank Katch of the University of Massachusetts, among many others, have compiled body composition data on elite athletes in a wide variety of sports from a number of studies. They identified an average body fat percentage among elite male marathon runners of just 3.3 percent—lower than in any other sport—and an average body fat percentage among female distance runners of 17.3 percent—lower than in every sport except bodybuilding and (of all things) modern pentathlon.

Your body fat level is also a good predictor of your running performance. A 2004 study from the University of Nebraska discovered an inverse correlation between body fat percentage and velocity at lactate threshold, meaning that leaner runners tended to run faster at lactate threshold intensity. Other research has found that body fat levels, specifically in the legs, predict performance among top-level runners. In other words, while all top-level runners are lean, the best of the best runners have the very leanest legs.

Why is body fat the enemy of running performance? A quick physiology lesson provides the answer. There are two basic categories of body fat: essential fat and storage fat. Essential fat is fat stored in bone marrow, the vital organs, and the muscles and tissues of the central nervous system. This fat provides insulation, protection, and energy for these organs and tissues and also aids in nerve signal transmission. It is termed "essential" because a certain minimum amount of fat in these organs and tissues is required for basic health. Storage fat, on the other hand, is fat contained in adipose tissue (specialized fat storage tissue), primarily in the abdomen in men and around the hips and buttocks in women, and, to a certain extent, underneath the skin in both sexes. This fat is a long-term energy reserve. When we eat more calories than we expend, we store the extra energy in this form. While useful in times of scarcity, storage fat is not essential for healthy functioning of the body, and too much of it increases the risk of chronic diseases such as high blood pressure and type 2 diabetes.

Essential fat comprises roughly 3 percent of the average man's body mass and about 12 percent of the average woman's body mass. Elite runners have about the same amount of essential fat as the rest of us but minimal

The Fat in Your Muscles

If you've ever fried a hamburger patty, you've seen liquid fat ooze out of the cooking meat and bubble on the hot skillet. That's because there is fat inside the muscles of cows—and there is fat inside your muscles, too. These fats are called intramuscular triglycerides, but you can just call them muscle fats.

Both muscle fats and free fatty acids (that is, fats in the bloodstream derived from adipose tissue) account for some of the energy contributed during running. The balance depends on the intensity and duration of the run and on the fitness level of the runner. Each runner is different, but we do know that the following three factors play a large role in determining how much fat you burn during exercise: genes, diet, and training status. Genes have the greatest influence in the equation. However, as you become more trained, your body learns to burn more fat at higher exercise intensities, as discussed in Chapter 8. In addition, eating a high-fat diet, while not so great for your health, has been proven to increase the amount of fat you burn during exercise.

amounts of storage fat. No advanced scientific measurement techniques are required to confirm this—simply observe the visible veins and muscles of elite long-distance runners as a sure sign of their low body fat percentage. This is the case in part because top runners are naturally (which is to say genetically) lean, but also because training incinerates excess storage fat, which is "dead weight" with respect to running. Since adipose tissue does not contribute to accomplishing work, it only adds to the energy cost of running. Yes, it is true that during running we will burn some fat, and the breakdown of storage fat provides energy, but even the leanest runner has more than enough storage fat to fuel the longest runs, as one pound of fat contains the equivalent of 4,000 calories, which could provide enough energy to power you for about five hours at a comfortable running speed.

The Right Amount of Fat

Just as high percentages of body fat will predispose you to cardiovascular disease, there is such a thing as being too lean. If there is not enough energy in the diet to maintain the body's essential fat, it will begin to degenerate, and a variety of health consequences will ensue: poor vitamin absorption, poor digestion, reduced HDL ("good") cholesterol, low energy, and, for runners, poor recovery from training, and even muscle loss. Excessive leanness is not rare among runners and is most common among female runners, but it almost always occurs as a result of disordered eating, exercise addiction, or both. Non-elite runners are more likely to have too much fat rather than too little for optimal performance.

Runners tend to struggle with their body fat levels these days for the same reasons that most nonrunners do. Evolution has given us bodies that are capable of storing energy efficiently, in the form of fat, for future use whenever we increase our food intake or reduce our activity level. This capability was beneficial in the past, but now it's a liability, because our modern lifestyle is much more sedentary than that of past generations and our diets are much more energy dense, making it easy to meet our daily caloric requirements but also easy to overindulge. This is a recipe for fat accumulation. Even most runners burn fewer calories each day than the average 18th-century farmer did. An interesting Canadian study found that Mennonite children—who shun modern conveniences such as televisions and cars—were more active thanks to the walking, bicycling, and chores they did as parts of their colonial-era lifestyle than their non-Mennonite peers, including those who played sports. They were also significantly leaner, fitter, and stronger.

Meanwhile, as our activity level has dropped, food intake has risen significantly in the United States over the past 30 years. This increase is widely believed to have been driven by increases in portion sizes of restaurant menu items and packaged foods, the result of competition among food businesses and substantial decreases in the cost of producing food.

The combination of portion size and the constant deluge of commercial advertising for food has essentially inflated our appetites—or created a breach between our physical and social appetites for food. Researchers, including consumer psychologist Brian Wansink of Cornell University, have shown that the amount of food we consume is strongly influenced by the accessibility of food, how much food is put in front of us, and social pressure to eat more, including pressure from commercial advertising. A perfect example of the latter influence is Taco Bell's invention of "fourth meal," a late-night fast-food meal that the television viewer is encouraged to add to his or her daily eating routine. Our pattern of food consumption has evolved (or devolved, as the case may be) and is now much more complex than simply eating when we are hungry.

While the leanest runners tend to be the best runners, and while most recreational runners are not as lean as they should be for optimal health, let alone optimal performance, there is no single body fat level that is best for every runner. In other words, not every runner is capable of becoming equally lean without compromising his or her health. Once again we have our parents to thank for this, because genetic factors are mostly responsible. One study found that body fat percentage is 64 percent inherited from one's parents. This means that if your parents have high levels of body fat, it's unlikely that you can become as lean as most elite runners are. Age is another factor. Visceral fat stores increase inexorably with age. "Body history" is yet another. If you've been severely overweight in the past, you might not be able to get as lean as you might otherwise. The situation is quite complex and multifactorial; if you desire to look like an elite marathon runner, be advised that it is most certainly *not* just a matter of dieting and running 100 miles per week.

How to Determine Your Optimal Body Composition

Given the fact that there is no one-size-fits-all body fat percentage, how can you determine the body fat percentage that is best for you? For runners, optimal body composition can be defined as the body fat level that is associated with maximal performance. In other words, the body fat percentage you have when you're in peak shape is likely to be your optimal body fat level. We must point out that body composition encompasses certain other measurable factors, such as muscle mass, lean mass, and even bone mass. But measurement of these factors is impossible without some specialized equipment and advanced equations that are not particularly accessible to most runners. For that reason, we discuss body composition with reference to body fat only.

The most precise way to determine your optimal body fat percentage is to create a graph that plots your body fat percentage against your performance over a long-term period of focused training (at least 12 months). The horizontal axis will define a range of body fat percentages that's a little broader than any fluctuations you're likely to experience throughout the year. The vertical axis will define a range of times from a recurring test workout that's a little broader than your performance fluctuations are likely to be over the course of a year. Once every four weeks, step on a body fat scale and note your body fat percentage. On the same day, perform a test workout that provides a good indicator of your race-specific fitness. For example, you might head down to the track and do a 10-K time trial at 95 percent effort.

Create a data point on the graph that represents your performance test result and body fat percentage on each test day. After you plot a few points, you will begin to notice a clear pattern. It is likely that you will achieve your best performance at your lowest body fat percentage. In any case, the body fat percentage at which you achieve your best performance represents your optimal body composition.

Repeatable Measurements

Without launching into a statistics lesson, it is important to note that when measuring something like body weight or body fat over time, you must know the variation of your equipment. This means that you have to know how much the measurement will change simply as a function of natural variation in the equipment. The problem is that if it is a highly variable device, then you will not be able to track changes over time; any changes you might measure will be less than the day-to-day variation of the equipment. Before starting your body fat and performance tracking, step on your analyzer scale once a day for 10 days and record the result each time. Be sure to take the measurement at the same time of day; probably when you wake up will be easiest. Plot these values on a simple graph to see how much the value changes. The key to understanding this is that we do not expect body fat percentage to change on a daily basis, and so any changes you see represent the equipment variation and not actual changes.

Feel free to track your actual body weight along with your body fat percentage, but use it as a secondary metric. Body fat percentage is more important. That's because you can reach any given body weight at more than one body fat percentage. For example, if you use smart training and healthy eating to reach a weight of 150 pounds, your body fat percentage (if you're male) might be 12. But if you use extreme dieting to reach the same weight, your body fat percentage might be 15, because you will have lost some muscle along with a little fat. As a result, you will underperform at this body weight. So tracking your body fat percentage along with your body weight can function as a check against making this mistake. Yes, you want to be light, but you don't want to be light at all costs. You want to be light and lean.

This table provides an example of the method of determining optimal body composition and weight that we just described. It presents the results of 5 testing days spread across 16 weeks of focused training (1 testing day every 4 weeks) that culminated in a peak race. The runner performed a 10-K run at 95 percent effort as her test workout and also measured her body weight and body fat percentage. The results show a clear trend toward better performance at lower body weights and body fat percentages.

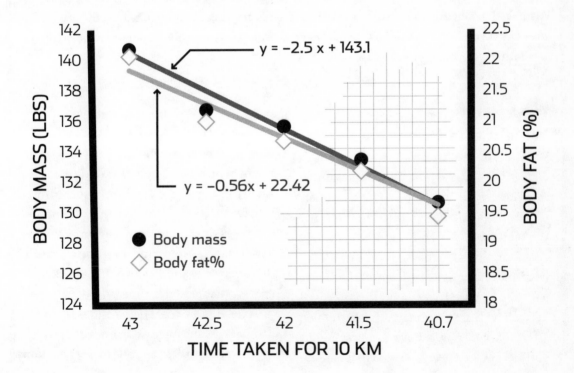

Measuring Leanness

Until recently, there was no affordable and convenient way for the average person to monitor his or her own body composition. Nowadays, body fat scales are available at pharmacies, department stores, and sporting goods stores. They cost about the same as a regular bathroom scale ($40 to $100), and they're just as easy to use. All you have to do is step on and read the numbers.

A body fat scale uses a technology called *bioelectrical impedance* to estimate body fat percentage. The device sends a weak electrical current into your body and measures the degree to which your body tissues resist it. Muscle impedes the current more than fat does. Bioelectrical impedance is not the most accurate way to measure body composition and is therefore not suitable for comparisons between individuals, but it does provide consistent results, so it is suitable for identifying trends within individuals. The most accurate measurement method is DEXA scanning, which is done only in clinical environments.

If you're already fairly lean, be sure to purchase a body fat scale with an "athlete mode," such as the Tanita Ironman. Units without this feature tend to be less accurate for athletes. Also, read the instructions that come with your body fat scale. Your results may be way off the mark if you fail to follow basic guidelines, such as emptying your bladder and moistening the bottoms of your feet before using the device.

How to Optimize Body Weight and Composition

What if you feel that you're still not lean enough even after several months of training consistently and trying to eat right? Runners often find themselves in this situation, and the method of determining optimal body composition that we have given you will not be of much use. Some runners' performance is limited by their very inability to reach optimal body fat percentage. If you are such a runner, you might have to pursue your optimal body fat level as a goal that is semi-independent of your goal to achieve optimal performance. In fact, we speak to athletes all the time who try to combine the two goals of performance and weight loss. This is a critical error, as you are doomed to suboptimal achievement in one or both areas. If improving both your body composition and your performance is important to you, then tackle one at a time, and keep your focus on one goal for that period of time.

Following are six basic ways to reduce your body weight and increase leanness. In practicing them, be sure to continue to pay attention to your running performance as a check against going too far. A drop in performance that happens despite sensible training and coincides with significant weight and/or fat loss indicates that you've shot past your optimal body composition—and if you've dropped below your optimal body composition for running performance, you've almost certainly also dropped below your ideal weight for maximum health.

INCREASE YOUR RUNNING VOLUME

Running more is one of the simplest and most effective ways to improve running performance. It is also one of the simplest and most effective ways to shed excess body fat. Of course, there is a limit to the maximum running volume before runners become injured or overtrained, but most runners are far from that threshold. More important is to implement short-term increases in volume, so that you don't ask too much of your body in too short a time. A small increase in running volume could make a measurable difference in your performance and body composition. For example, if you currently run an average of 40 miles per week, you might increase your training volume to 50 miles per week, carefully adding 5 miles each week over two weeks so as not to overdo it. This change will add only 10 to 12 minutes to your daily exercise burden, yet it will result in burning an extra 800 to 1,400 calories each week.

The 10 percent per week guideline provides a typically safe increase in running volume. Guidelines rarely work for *everyone*, however, so listen to your body and cut back for a few days whenever you experience intensifying fatigue or sore areas. Avoid trying to pack too many miles into each run. If you currently run fewer than five times per week, start by adding another short run to your weekly routine, and then another if necessary, until you're running 6 days a week. Then start adding distance to one or more existing runs, if you wish.

If you believe that you are already running as much as your body can handle, you still might be able to burn additional calories without overtraining by adding cross-training workouts such as bicycling to your weekly routine. Such activities burn comparable amounts of calories to running but do not subject the lower extremities to additional pounding. Feel free to do as much as one cross-training workout for every run you do (building gradually to that level, of course). There is precedent for this approach, even in the elite ranks. For example, in the middle of his career, 2004 Olympic Marathon silver medalist Meb Keflezighi switched to a new training schedule in which he bicycled as often as he ran. His goal was not to shed excess body fat but to reduce his injury risk without sacrificing fitness; nevertheless, he set a good example for runners who want to get leaner but prefer not to take the risk of running more.

INCREASE YOUR RUNNING INTENSITY

Back in the 1920s, the legendary British exercise physiologist A. V. Hill first observed that the body's rate of oxygen consumption remains elevated for some time after exercise and that this phenomenon is indicative of a metabolic rate that, while lower than the metabolic rate during exercise itself, remains above the normal resting metabolic rate. This phenomenon has come to be known as excess postexercise oxygen consumption (EPOC). More recent research has determined that EPOC has two phases: a strong acute phase lasting up to 2 hours and a weaker long-term phase lasting 24 hours or more, the sum of which accounts for 6 to 15 percent of the total caloric cost of a workout, depending on its duration and intensity. Thus, if you burn 1,000 calories during a workout, you can expect to burn roughly an extra 100 calories in excess of your normal resting metabolism in the hours after the workout.

Different types of workouts produce different levels of EPOC. High-intensity cardiovascular exercise (think interval sessions) result in the largest amounts of postexercise energy consumption. Indeed, EPOC increases exponentially at exercise intensities exceeding roughly 60 percent of VO_2 max. Exercise scientists who performed the earliest studies on the effects of high-intensity intermittent exercise on body weight and composition were shocked by the results. A recent study from the University of New South Wales, Australia, found that women lost an average of 10.5 percent of their fat mass after 15 weeks on a three-times-a-week program of 20-minute workouts consisting of 8-second stationary bike sprints followed by 12-second passive recoveries. (Sounds easy, but that's 60 all-out sprints—a hellishly hard workout, so don't be fooled!) Subjects in a control group that performed traditional endurance workouts lost considerably less fat over the same period despite spending roughly 400 percent more time pedaling.

High-intensity intervals are not only great fat burners but are also terrific fitness builders. For example, in a study conducted by researchers at the University of Cape Town, South Africa, trained cyclists significantly improved their time trial performances by incorporating six workouts of 30-second sprint repeats into their training over a three-week period.

Many runners underutilize high-intensity training. Your weekly regimen should include two high-intensity runs per week—usually one set of intervals (such as 10 x 400 meters at 1500-meter race pace with 400-meter jogging recoveries) and a tempo run (such as 30 minutes at threshold pace)—in addition to a few easy runs. Increasingly, competitive runners follow this type of schedule year-round, instead of concentrating their high-intensity work in the weeks immediately preceding races. If you're currently doing fewer than two high-intensity runs per week or are not doing high-intensity running during the off-season and base-building periods, you will undoubtedly experience improvements in your body composition and performance by correcting this training imbalance. As for training volume, however, don't make any rapid changes and suddenly introduce two high-intensity workouts per week—you're headed for disaster by doing this. Rather, spend a month working those sessions into the program—adding faster running is one of the riskiest parts of the program, so do it with caution! Finally, the amount of high-intensity running you do should decrease during the off-season and base-building phases—but don't phase it out entirely.

BE MORE CONSISTENT

Very few runners stay at the same body weight all year. It is normal for runners to gain some weight in the winter off-season when they are training less. But some runners let themselves go too much at this time of year, not only training less but also eating more because of holiday temptations. As a result, they put on more extra fat than they can take off during the rest of the year. Research suggests that the average American adult gains two pounds during the six weeks between Thanksgiving and New Year's Eve and never loses them. The same happens all over the world. It is not for nothing that one of the most common New Year's resolutions is

to lose the weight that has been added in the preceding three weeks! Runners are less likely to gain permanent weight through the holidays, but reduced activity and increased eating may prevent them from ever reaching their optimal body composition in the race season.

To avoid this situation, try to maintain consistent training and eating habits throughout the year. While it is beneficial to reduce your training somewhat in the off-season to give your body a chance to regenerate, it is not beneficial to "slack off." Continue to get some exercise daily, even if it's in alternative activities such as cross-country skiing or indoor cycling. And while there's no harm in pigging out on holidays and at the office holiday party, there *is* potential harm in snacking on Christmas cookies daily between special occasions. Research from the National Weight Control Registry has shown that men and women who maintain consistent eating habits throughout the year are much less likely to regain previously lost weight. So eat the same on December 29 as you do on July 17—assuming you eat right on July 17!

MATCH CALORIE INTAKE TO CALORIE EXPENDITURE

Usually—but not always—runners who have a hard time shedding those last few pounds to achieve their optimal body fat percentage are consistently eating more calories than their bodies use each day. And in most cases, it's because they're eating more than they think they are. Research has shown that people commonly underestimate how much they eat by as much as 20 percent. By taking the time to estimate your daily calorie needs and count your calorie intake, you can find out whether you've been eating more than you think you have and take steps to balance calories in and calories out.

Your daily calorie needs are determined by your resting metabolic rate (or RMR, which is determined primarily by your lean body mass) and the number of calories you burn through running. The formulas used to make these calculations are fairly complex, so we recommend that you use an online calculator (such as the one at www.shapeup.org) to do the work for you. All you have to do is enter your height, weight, age, and gender, and the calculator spits out an estimated number of calories your body uses each day at rest. For example, if you are a 40-year-old woman who stands 5'6" and weights 130 pounds, the calculator at shapeup.org will tell you that your RMR is 1,272 calories. This is just a prediction, but these formulas are sufficiently accurate for your use, as most have been validated in the laboratory.

The next step is to calculate how many additional calories you burn each day through activity. There are online calculators for this, as well. If you enter your weight and a specific duration, these calculators tell you roughly how many calories you burn in various activities (and at various intensities, in some cases) in that amount of time. Let's suppose that on a typical day, our hypothetical 40-year-old woman who stands 5'6" and weights 130 pounds runs for 45 minutes at a pace of 9 minutes per mile and also takes her dog for a brisk 20-minute walk, and that's about it in terms of activity. According to one online calculator, she burns about 487.5 calories during her run and 75 more on her walk. Add these numbers to her RMR to get a total calorie expenditure of approximately 1,834.5 calories per day. Note that it does not take into account the elevated metabolic rate after exercise, which we discussed previously. However, given that these equations are only estimates and not 100 percent accurate, that level of detail is probably self-defeating anyway. Be aware of it, but don't obsess too much over it.

The next step is to estimate the number of food calories consumed each day. To do this, record in a journal everything you eat and drink for three days. Try to include one weekend day, as often we eat differently (i.e., more!) at social events. Use food labels and resources such as nutritiondata.com to get accurate calorie counts. Add up the total number of calories consumed each day and find the average for the three days. This number should be roughly equal to your estimate of energy expenditure from one of the online calculators. Note that it is impossible to be 100 percent accurate in doing this. Your margins of error are necessarily large, because it's not possible to measure calories burned or calories consumed with a high degree of resolution. So accept that this is a guideline, not a scale that you have to balance. The only outcome of the latter approach is that you'll stress yourself into weight loss!

However, as a guide, this kind of knowledge is useful. If, for example, your calorie intake is significantly greater than your output, then you know that your difficulty in shedding that excess body fat probably stems from too much eating. So now what do you do? Look back at your food journals. Somewhere in there you are bound to find some waste—some food and beverage choices that contribute calories to your daily total without adding nutrition. Eliminate or cut back on these calorie inflators or find lower-calorie substitutes for them. For example, replace your 16-ounce morning caffe latte with a cup of lightly sweetened green tea, eliminate the potato chips from your lunch, or replace your evening bowl of ice cream with a single bite of dark chocolate or a cup of low-fat yogurt. After making these changes, count your daily calories again.

One study found that dieters who kept a regular food journal lost twice as much weight as dieters who followed the same program but did not keep a journal. Simply going through the exercise of balancing your calories in and calories out will make you more mindful of what and how much you eat and encourage you to control your diet more carefully.

EAT MORE PROTEIN

High-protein diets—in which protein provides as much as 30 percent of daily calories—have lately caught the interest of nutrition and obesity researchers, who have found that such diets reduce hunger and preserve muscle mass during caloric restriction. This evidence suggests that it may be beneficial for individuals seeking to lose weight to increase their protein consumption at the same time they reduce their daily calorie intake; by doing so they may be more likely to remain on the diet (due to reduced hunger) and may lose more fat and less muscle.

If you're struggling to shed those last few pounds of flab through your normal training and eating habits, you might want to consider making at least a short-term shift to a higher-protein diet. You can do this in a healthy way by eating more fish, poultry, lean meats, eggs, and low-fat dairy foods. In some studies, protein shakes have also been used to increase protein intake in a calorically efficient manner. When you make the transition, keep a food journal for a few days and analyze it to make sure your protein intake reaches 25 to 30 percent of total calories.

Although most of the studies on the effects of a high-protein diet on body weight and composition have involved a planned reduction in total calories, some studies have found that people automatically eat fewer calories on high-protein diets, which are so filling. As a runner, you might fare best on a high-protein diet if you do not consciously cut back on total calories, because combining increased protein intake with a significant calorie reduction might wreak havoc on your running. The only way to increase protein intake and reduce calorie intake simultaneously is to sharply reduce your consumption of fat and/or carbohydrate, which are better energy sources than protein.

Few runners consciously maintain a high-protein diet. However, there are some examples of high-performing runners who eat a relatively high-protein diet. Among them is Dean Karnazes, winner of the 2004 Badwater Ultramarathon, who claims to follow a classic "Zone Diet" comprising roughly 40 percent carbohydrate, 30 percent fat, and 30 percent protein. Six-time Hawaii Ironman winner Mark Allen followed the same diet throughout his career. There is some question about whether the intent of these athletes matches reality. It is difficult to maintain such a diet with anything resembling normal meal choices, which gives doubters cause for speculation that runners and other athletes on Zone-type diets eat less protein and more carbohydrate than they think they do. Remember, however, that attempting to follow a diet that is totally impractical will likely result in failure to lose weight, improve body composition, or improve running performance. So choose your approach wisely.

Very little research on the effects of high protein intake on endurance performance has been done. In one short-term study, New Zealand researchers found that cycling time trial performance was significantly impaired after 7 days on a high-protein diet. The diet in this study derived 30 percent of calories from protein, which is three times the minimum daily requirement of 10 percent. If you find your running performance to be impaired after 10 or more days on a high-protein diet, abandon it and turn your focus toward other ways of getting lighter and leaner.

PRACTICE NUTRIENT TIMING

Another reason for difficulty in achieving one's optimal competitive weight is poor nutrient timing. *When* you eat is almost as important as *what* you eat, because the same nutrients have different effects on the body when consumed at different times. The body's energy needs fluctuate throughout the day. It's important to concentrate your food intake during those times when your body's energy needs are greatest and not to consume more calories than your body needs to meet its immediate energy needs at any time. When you consume calories at times of peak energy need, most of them are used to fuel your muscles and nervous system, to synthesize muscle tissue, and to replenish muscle fuel stores. When you consume more calories than you need at any time, those excess calories will be stored as body fat.

Even consuming too few calories at times of peak energy needs could make you less lean by switching your body chemistry into a fat-storing mode. This was shown in a study involving elite female gymnasts and distance runners, which found a strong inverse relationship between the number and size of energy deficits throughout the day (that is, periods when the body's calorie needs exceed the calorie supply from foods) and body fat percentage. In other words, the athletes who did the best job of matching their calorie intake with their calorie needs throughout the day were leaner than those who tended to fall behind.

What's important to note about this study is that the effect of mini-calorie deficits was independent of total caloric intake for the day. This means that an athlete who requires and consumes x calories a day is likely to have less muscle and more body fat if she does not time her eating well than if she takes in the same total number of calories but distributes them more evenly throughout the day.

A simple example of this from the scientific literature is that individuals who skip breakfast weigh more than those who eat breakfast regularly. Eventually, at some point in the day, the breakfast skippers more than make up for the missed calories at the start of their day. Consuming inadequate calories early in the day and failing to eat in the first hour after workouts, when energy needs are high, as well as eating large meals late in the day, are factors that are associated with higher body weights and higher body fat levels. For example, a Japanese study found that boxers placed on a six-meals-a-day weight-control diet lowered their body fat percentage significantly more than boxers who ate exactly the same number of calories in just two meals. An eating frequency of five to six meals per day is optimal for athletes. That's because by dividing the total number of calories you need each day into five or six allotments, you will better avoid small energy deficits, and each meal and snack is small enough to avoid consuming excess calories in any single meal that wind up being stored as body fat.

The most important time to eat is within the first hour after exercise. Your body needs calories to replenish muscle fuel stores and rebuild damaged muscle tissues at this time. By consuming a good portion of your day's calories in the postexercise period, you ensure that these calories are used almost entirely to support your muscles instead of being stored as body fat. Studies have shown that athletes who take in adequate nutrition after workouts build more muscle and lose more fat than those who ingest exactly the same total amount and types of calories during the entire day but who fail to consume any of these calories during the first two hours after workouts.

There's no need to force yourself to eat more than you're hungry for after exercise. Just get in the habit of consuming a comfortable amount of carbohydrates and protein

Recovery Meals

Breakfast

Egg white omelet with tomatoes, peppers, onions, and mushrooms

Toast with blueberry jam

Large glass of orange juice

Lunch

Turkey sandwich with lettuce and mustard on whole grain bread

Banana

Large glass of apple juice

Dinner

Spaghetti with tomato sauce and meatballs (lean beef or turkey)

Garden salad with olive oil and vinegar dressing

Glass of water

from healthy sources, along with fluid for rehydration, of course. Above are three examples of good post workout meals.

The Long View

Even if you do everything right, you will probably never be as lean as the likes of Paula Radcliffe and Haile Gebrselassie. Although your extra insulation may be one factor that prevents you from running as fast as the world's best runners, achieving your personal optimal body composition will help you become the best runner you can be—and will confer other benefits. As we mentioned, though, you have your parents to thank for most of this, and on that note, it is important to come to grips with your own body, regardless of how much or how little body fat it carries. You can be the most diligent runner and dieter out there, but eventually you will reach an optimal level, and if that level is not the 6 percent you desire, then you must try to accept your body and love it for what it does for you—which is provide you with a vehicle to enjoy running!

The average American gains a pound or two of body fat every year from the beginning of adulthood through middle age. These accumulating fat stores compromise health in a variety of well-known ways. This pattern has become so common that it is widely considered normal, but it isn't. Runners tend to gain significantly less weight and body fat than their sedentary counterparts. Indeed, a 1998 study found that postmenopausal female runners were no heavier than female runners in their late 20s, and their body fat percentages were still significantly lower than those of sedentary young women.

The race of life is one that none of us wants to finish first. Pursuing your optimal body composition will help you "lose" this race by staying physiologically younger longer and by slowing down less as you age.

The Central Ne

rvous System

The "final frontier" in the pursuit of human performance. . . . For some reason, that description is true as applied to the central nervous system. It seems difficult to believe, because we all know that the brain (or what we tend to oversimplify as the *mind,* as we'll see shortly) is crucial to our running performance. But it seems that the scientific community has only just awakened to the fact that running, like everything else, starts and ends in the brain.

Perhaps the scientists should have asked a runner for perspective on the importance of the brain during exercise. Every single one of you will have experienced the battle that rages in your mind during your hard training sessions or races. That battle, the struggle between what you perceive as mind versus matter, is clearly pivotal to your quest to become a better runner. Yet science traditionally neglected the role of this organ in determining our performance ability. That is not so much the result of a failure to recognize the brain's importance as it is the near impossibility of trying to understand this incredibly complex system. Consequently, theories such as the concept that a VO_2 max and muscle fiber type limit your ability to run were developed without ever giving much consideration to this bothersome organ!

That is one extreme. At the other, we tend to oversimplify this vastly complex interaction between the brain and our physiological systems by reducing the discussion to "mind over matter." This is a huge oversimplification because it neglects to acknowledge that everything, from the signal that tells your muscles to contract, to the increase in your heart rate, to the signal that's sent to your liver to start converting glycogen to glucose so that your muscles have fuel to burn, originates in the brain. Therefore, performance is possible thanks to the *physiology* that is controlled by the brain. So, too, the latest insights suggest that performance is limited or regulated by those same *physiological* processes.

Perhaps the newest branch of exercise physiology is the study of the role of the brain in determining fatigue. Some revolutionary theories have been proposed, and have challenged the paradigm that fatigue and the limits to performance reside in the muscle. Instead, it's the brain that is now recognized as holding the key to unlocking hidden running potential through its regulation of pacing strategies and the amount of muscle that you can activate when you run. Unlock the secrets of the brain, and you'll be a better runner. Unfortunately, it's not that easy, and we may be many years away—if

ever—from fully unlocking or tapping into this reserve. After all, your brain probably serves a protective function during exercise, and overriding this may not be in your body's best interests. We'll look at these considerations in detail in Chapter 11 as we discuss the role of the brain in fatigue.

We'll also address the issue of running technique. Since the brain initiates muscle contraction, our running technique is in no small part a function of how the brain coordinates muscle activation. One of the livelier debates among running communities is whether technique should be learned as skill or allowed to develop naturally without specific technique training.

Finally, the mind-body link is so intricately related that our emotional response to running has physiological underpinnings. The concept of a "runner's high," presumed to be the result of endorphin release during exercise—but probably more complex than this—is familiar to all and experienced by many. We run for the health benefits, the goal orientation, and the challenges it provides, but now recognize that our psychological, emotional, and even spiritual well-being are part of the package.

[Chapter 11]

Mind Matter over Body Matter

In October 2008, Haile Gebrselassie, arguably the greatest distance runner ever, broke his own marathon world record, clocking 2:03:59 on the streets of Berlin. One year earlier, he had broken perennial rival Paul Tergat's mark of 2:04:55, also in Berlin. The end result was that within only one year, the world record had fallen by almost a minute, and the 2:04 barrier had been broken. As is typical after a world record is broken, the world began looking ahead to the next barrier, and many observers of the sport jumped on the idea that man will one day run a sub-2-hour marathon. David Bedford, the organizer of the London Marathon, stated that he was positive he'd see a sub-2-hour performance in his lifetime. Others are not quite as sure, suggesting that he might need to live another 100 years for that to be remotely possible.

Regardless of who turns out to be right, it's a fun debate. The presence of barriers, the physiology of breaking them, and the limits to performance are fascinating topics to discuss, and they are what this chapter is all about.

Perhaps the best example of barrier busting in athletic history dates back to 1954: the culmination of the chase for the 4-minute mile. This is a story that is probably familiar to you. The world mile record was broken four times between 1931 and 1942. In 1942, it stood at 4:06.4 but fell rapidly, thanks to six records in three years by the great Swedish runners Arne Andersson and Gunder Hägg. By 1945, when World War II ended, the mile record was 4:01.4, tantalizingly close to the 4-minute barrier. Everyone expected that it was a matter of time before someone would run a mile in under 4 minutes. But for the next nine years, the record was not broken, let alone taken under 4 minutes. There are extenuating circumstances, though—world war deprived the sport of many of its potential runners, and there was an inevitable lull in performance immediately after the war ended.

By 1951, a new crop of talent, including Australia's John Landy, England's Roger Bannister, and an American named Wes Santee, had begun their quest to break 4 minutes. John Landy was the frontrunner—between 1952 and 1954, he ran between 4:02 and 4:03 no less than six times. In one famous race in December 1953, he needed only to run the final 220 yards in 30.6 seconds to break the 4-minute barrier, but he tied up in the final straight, finishing in 4:02. After this race, Landy famously declared to a group of reporters, "I feel I could go on for 10 years, but I don't think it's worth it. *Frankly, I think the 4-minute mile is beyond my capabilities* [our emphasis]. Two seconds may not sound much, but to me it's like trying to break through a brick wall. Someone may achieve the 4-minute mile the world is wanting so desperately, but I don't think I can."

Then, on May 6, 1954, at the Iffley Road track in Oxford, England, Roger Bannister set off with the assistance of two pace runners and proceeded to run himself into history, with a mile time of 3:59.4. He had done it; he won the race and a permanent place in athletic legend. But the story does not end there. Forty-six days later, John Landy smashed the record by running 3:57.9, an incredible 4 seconds faster than he'd ever run before. Remem-

ber that this is a man who said that the 4-minute barrier was a brick wall, and he found a 2-second improvement impossible for two years! Landy's statement is often taken as his admission of defeat, which is probably a little harsh. More likely, he was simply deflecting some of the pressure, and he still believed he was capable of breaking 4 minutes. However, the point is that once Bannister did it, Landy followed, with a much greater improvement on the performance than he probably even considered possible before.

The physiological question is not necessarily what did Bannister do to run sub–4 minutes (though this is of course important and worth consideration), but rather which physiological factors can possibly explain how Landy could improve by 4 seconds in the space of 5 months, having battled for 3 years to find 2 seconds? It seems unlikely that training, lactate threshold, VO_2 max, or any other measurable physiological parameter (at least that we know of) can explain this change in so short a time. You could probably attribute his improvement to the removal of a mental barrier, and that seems reasonable; Landy needed the "brick wall" to be broken down for him, and that's what Bannister did.

However, now you have to ask the following question: When Landy was busy reeling off his six 4:02 performances, why could he not go faster? In that race where he was within sight of the record with only 200 meters to go, why did he tie up and fail to hold his pace? In hindsight, you'd blame the mental barrier, but at the time, it would probably have been put down to excessive lactate poisoning the muscles, insufficient oxygen being delivered to the muscles, or some other failure that prevented his muscles from doing their job, causing him to lose those valuable 2 seconds. As you read this, you may be in a similar situation. Whenever you run up against a seemingly insurmountable limit in your efforts to get faster in training or racing, you will also probably blame these factors. But to suggest that Landy's performance improved thanks to the removal of the mental barrier would imply that whatever physiological limits existed before were either overridden (a possibility) or insignificant all along. That seems implausible.

Put it this way: If the performance limit existed solely in the muscles, the heart, or the metabolic system, then finding 4 seconds of improvement thanks to the breaking down of a mental "wall" is impossible to explain. If, however, physiology was always linked to the mental component, then you can appreciate how a change in mental state could influence the physiological performance. This, of course, means that none of these physiological systems were truly "limiting" to begin with, though they are certainly significant, as we shall see. This interaction between the the mind and the body is a fascinating and poorly understood area of exercise science.

Mind over Matter? Or Matter of a Different Kind?

The old adage "mind over matter" is a quasi-philosophical concept that is thrown around with abandon. The notion that pure, non-physical "mind" is able to somehow defy physical laws as they are manifest in the workings of the body is a massive oversimplification of the truth and is, quite honestly, more than likely incorrect. Just as you cannot commit suicide by holding your breath, you have to realize that you cannot simply "believe" yourself into becoming a world-class runner. Physiology always wins the day. John Landy did not suddenly break 3:58 because he gained a belief that enabled him to run beyond his true physical limits. He possessed the abilities all along; he just needed a final piece of the puzzle to fall into place, and Bannister provided it. Therefore, we must emphasize that when we talk about the role of the brain in your running, we are not limiting ourselves to psychology. The adage should in fact be "brain matter over body matter," because as we develop our understanding of the integration between the brain and the physiological systems, we realize that the regulation of performance is a complex result of how all these systems interact, comparable to the body as an orchestra, with the brain as its conductor.

Because of their rather conceptual nature, theories of the role of the brain in determining performance have received much criticism. Part of the problem is that it is virtually impossible to measure brain function (especially emotional and cognitive processes during exercise) with the same accuracy as we can measure blood lactate levels, glucose concentrations, VO_2 max values, and heart rates. It is perhaps for this reason that the role of the brain in determining athletic performance has been so underappreciated—it is simply too complex to appreciate.

The same Roger Bannister who ran himself into history with his 3:59.4 time would go on to become a world-renowned neurosurgeon (coincidentally studying the very organ that we will see was crucial to his success). He once remarked, "The human body is centuries in advance of the physiologist and can perform an integration of heart, lungs, and muscles which is too complex for the scientist to analyze."

Not to be too discouraged by that statement, let's begin to analyze just how the "conductor" integrates all the systems of its orchestra.

Fatigue as a Failure of Physiology

Ever since scientists first began studying the body during exercise, there has been a belief that fatigue occurs because the system fails— it fails to provide energy, fails to supply oxygen, fails to get rid of heat, fails to dispel "poisonous" metabolic products like lactate, and so on. You are probably at least somewhat familiar with concepts, such as oxygen debt,

anaerobic threshold, lactate accumulation, glycogen depletion, and heatstroke, used to explain why you slow down or feel tired when you run fast or far enough to test your limits.

For example, the oxygen limitation model holds that if you run too fast, your heart and lungs are unable to supply the oxygen that your active muscles require. Consequently, your muscles become anaerobic and accumulate lactate and hydrogen ions, causing the acidity level of the muscle to rise and eventually leading to that heavy-legged, burning sensation that forces you to slow down. Or how about the theory that you become fatigued and slow down because your muscles run out of glycogen, their most valuable source of energy? Then there is the theory that under certain conditions, you have to reduce speed because your body has failed to dissipate the heat that your working muscles produce, and your body temperature has risen dangerously high. The common thread in all these theories is that failure leads to fatigue—you slow down because one of your systems (or instruments, to continue the orchestra analogy) breaks down and fails to keep your body in homeostasis.

There is certainly a great deal of value and elements of truth in these theories, but they are the result of some rather unnatural research, that asks, "Why do athletes eventually *stop* exercising?" In order to answer this question, scientists make athletes do unnatural exercise trials, such as running on a treadmill at the same speed until they simply give up and can no longer keep moving—quite literally a "run-till-you-drop" approach. Thanks to this kind of study, we know that when your body temperature hits a cutoff point (which happens to be about 104°F), you stop. That is the point at which the failure of thermoregulation has been observed.

These studies made a huge contribution to our understanding of what actually happens at the point when we are forced to halt exercise. The problem is that these "limiting" or "critical" failure points have been offered as an explanation for why you slow down in real-world circumstances such as races, where there is an option between continuing at your original pace and stopping completely. In other words, it is contended that you slow down in the marathon because you don't have enough energy left or have become too hot or exceeded your anaerobic threshold.

The Pacing Strategy and Fatigue

But slowing down is not the same as stopping. This is obvious. Think of your last 10-K race (or your next one). Do you go out and run at a certain pace until you stop? Do you intend to run at, say, six minutes per mile until you are forced to stop and just hope that this comes after the finish line of the race? Of course not! So what the classic studies on the causes of exercise fatigue fail to recognize is that exercise is never one-paced. You are never forced

to speed up or prevented from slowing down. Of course, pride, competitive spirit, and race situations may drive you to harder efforts than you should be making (efforts which you will sooner or later pay back with interest!), but you always have an option to slow down (or speed up) if you need to.

So what are the implications of being able to adjust your pace? Well, that ability is the foundation of a key concept called the pacing strategy. Your pacing strategy is nothing more than the way you attempt to distribute your energy reserves over the course of a race. There is not a runner alive who has not made the error of going out too hard, only to pay back doubly in the second half of the race. And we have all run conservatively, often reaping the benefits of our restraint later in the race, when we glide past tired runners who seem to have reached their physiological limits.

Despite every runner's familiarity with the pacing experience, until relatively recently there was no known physiological explanation for pacing strategies. For example, if we assume for a second that fatigue occurs because the muscles are weakened by a chemical such as lactate, then as lactate levels get higher and higher over the course of a race, our running speeds should decrease. The paradox, however, is that most runners speed up in the final stretch of most races, even though lactate levels are at their highest then. This "end spurt" phenomenon, an impossibility according to the classic model

(*continued on page 192*)

Pacing like a Pro: How Elite Runners Pace Themselves

In considering your pacing strategy in a race, you can probably recall an occasion when you entered the final few hundred meters of a race and suddenly discovered speed in your legs that two minutes earlier you had thought was nonexistent. Your legs felt tired and empty, and you were fighting with all your strength to keep moving. Chances are, you started the race quickly, then slowed down at least slightly, despite consciously giving it your all during the middle kilometers. Yet once that finish line appeared in the distance, your spring returned, and you finished with a flurry of newfound energy.

The more critical analysts would say that you had paced yourself badly, because the fact that you could speed up meant that you did not use all your energy during the race—you left something on the road, so your pacing was not optimal. They say that you should finish with no reserve whatsoever. And certainly, if you have a superhuman sprint finish in you, it's likely that you did leave too much in reserve. But is this "end spurt" really a sign of suboptimal pacing? That's debatable, but you can take comfort from the fact that about 60 world record holders have experienced it too.

The accompanying graph shows the average kilometer time for every one of the 32 men's 5000-meter world records and 34 men's 10,000-meter world records ever set. The pattern is probably like your own racing strategy (whether executed consciously or not): fast start, slow progressively in the middle, and finish very fast, with the fastest kilometer of the race almost always coming right at the end. When the final kilometer is not the fastest, almost invariably the first kilometer is: In 26 world records at 10,000 meters, only once has any kilometer other than the first or final kilometer been the quickest.

Interestingly, it also appears that this typical pattern may be changing subtly. If you break the world records down into different eras, you find that the more recent records display a much more constant pacing strategy. They still have the fastest kilometer at the end, but the pronounced slowing of pace during the middle kilometers seems to be disappearing. So instead of starting fast, slowing down, and then finishing very fast, the pattern over the past 20 years has been to start fast, run fast in the middle, and then finish very fast.

This may result from training or from the fact that the African runners (who have set all of the records of the past 20 years) possess some physiological gift that allows them to adopt a different pacing strategy from those previously seen (which would partly explain why African runners dominate the long-distance events). Regardless, it does suggest that your objective for "optimal pacing" is not necessarily to finish without that end spurt—the spurt is normal. However, you also need to focus on preventing too much of a drop in pace in the middle kilometers, as we've seen the African runners achieve in recent times.

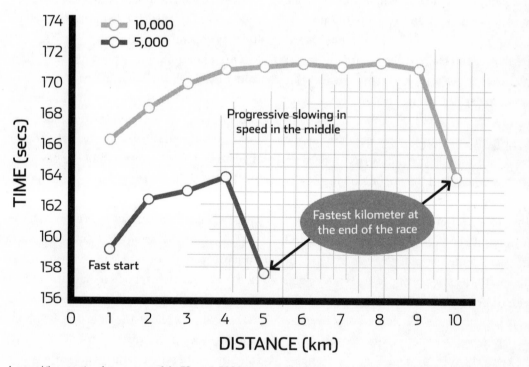

Average kilometer time for every one of the 32 men's 5000-meter world records and 34 men's 10,000-meter world records

of exercise fatigue, is evident in runners of all ability levels. In fact, in every single one of the 26 world records ever set in the men's 10,000 meters, the middle kilometers were the slowest and the final kilometer was the fastest of the race. It is a safe bet that the same is true of your own 5-K, 10-K, or marathon personal bests. (Well, maybe not the marathon!)

The Pacing Paradox

So what does it all mean? Practically, it means that you do not slow down simply because your muscles can't do their job anymore. If this were the case, you would never be able to speed up again. It also means that fatigue and the limits to exercise performance are a lot harder to define than was originally thought. Instead, we have a very complex pacing strategy, which forces us to slow down when we could speed up and then allows us to speed up when we should (in theory) be slowing down.

Recently, scientists at the University of Cape Town have been at the forefront of a revolution in thought about exercise performance and have contributed several novel approaches, or models, to the science of pacing strategy and exercise performance. The model in which the brain contributes to the regulation of exercise was developed by Professor Tim Noakes. Called the central governor model, or the complex systems model, for performance, it aims to explain how we exercise when we can choose to speed up and slow down as we please.

Pacing: Controlled by the Brain to Protect the Body

The most obvious and easy-to-understand example of a pacing strategy comes from studies of exercise in the heat. The "run-till-you-drop" study method showed that you eventually stop running at a body temperature of about 104°F—this is the limit. Remarkably, goats, mice, dogs, and even cheetahs stop at similar temperatures, suggesting that there is a "short-circuit" type of physiology, in which a critically high brain temperature causes a sudden failure to activate muscle and thus forces the animal to stop, even when its life may depend on continuing.

This phenomenon is perhaps best illustrated by the hunting strategy of the Khoi people, who live in the hot and dry conditions of the Kalahari Desert, living off the land and hunting for food. They have realized that if they hunt in the hottest part of the day (over 110°F), the animals they chase can run only for a limited time before they literally overheat and have to stop running. This is because the larger animals, which do not share our human capacity to lose heat by sweating, experience a faster rise in body temperature than we do. (We will see shortly how size is crucial in the heat.) Therefore, the Khoi people simply run slowly after the animal for hours in searing-hot temperatures until the animal lies down, unable to continue moving.

During running, however, our situation is not quite as dire as this. We have the capacity to speed up and the option to slow down, and we usually also know how long our exercise bout will last. And when you allow for these factors in a laboratory study, then a different picture emerges.

That picture reveals that you pace yourself given the known exercise duration and your "conductor's" ability to coordinate and respond to all the changes in physiology that occur during exercise. A few years ago, one of us (Ross) performed a study in which cyclists rode 20-kilometer time trials in an environmental chamber in both hot (95°F) and cool (50°F) conditions. The study found that the cyclists slowed down in the heat, even though they were not actually hotter than in the cool condition. Intuitively, one would expect that in the heat, the cyclists would get hotter and would thus slow down. Instead, they simply started the 20-kilometer trials at a lower power output and remained slower through the trials in the hot condition. As a result, their performance was slower, but they did not overheat. You may think this is obvious, but remember that the scientific theory—the textbook knowledge—is that you slow down because you are hot. This not true! Rather, it's a case of *slowing down so that you don't overheat.* In other words, it is a matter of "anticipatory regulation" of physiology through the adjustment of performance.

How were physiology and performance actually controlled? Well, we found that a lesser amount of muscle was activated by the brain in the hot condition than in the cool condition. This means that the brain actually "decided" to use less muscle right from the beginning, and, as a result, the athletes went slower in the heat.

Ask the question, What if the cyclists did not slow down? Their body temperature would rise and rise until they hit the limit of 104°F, and then they'd be forced to stop completely. Obviously, if you are racing or doing a time trial, stopping early is failure. Instead, the brain makes us slow down *before* this happens so we can sustain a steady level of performance all the way to the finish So now we see how the brain conducts the orchestra, activating muscle at just the right level so that we can exercise safely without overheating. This is why Professor Noakes coined the term "the central governor," giving a name to the organ that seemed to "govern," or regulate, everything that is happening during exercise.

The problem is that we still don't really know how the brain does this. Sure, we know that it simply forces us to use less muscle and therefore to slow down, but how? The answer probably lies in a concept called teleoanticipation.

Teleoanticipation

Teleoanticipation is a word that literally means "end anticipation." It was first used by the German scientist H. V. Ulmer, who came up with the theory that the brain takes into consideration the finishing point of exercise in ways that we are not consciously aware of.

More specifically, the brain uses this awareness to calculate how fast you can run (in the case of running) without bonking before the end point and then encourages you to speed up or slow down, based on the results of these calculations.

The key here is feedback—the rest of the body must tell the brain how it is doing. All those potentially limiting factors we mentioned earlier—muscle glycogen levels, oxygen levels, body temperature, metabolites—are communicated to the brain, so that it knows what our physiological status is. Our pacing strategy is determined by how the brain interprets what is going on in the body in the overall context of this known end point. Alan St. Clair Gibson, a professor of exercise science in Newcastle, England, has extended this concept to include "anchor points." These include where you start, where you finish, and where you are at any given moment in relation to these points.

So let's apply this concept to an athlete running a 10-K race. He starts the race, knowing that it is exactly 10 kilometers long and he is usually able to finish in 45 minutes (his goal and end point—two "anchors"). However, assume that it's a very hot and humid day, which means his goal of 45 minutes may be physiologically unattainable. If he does not adjust his early pace and runs at a 45-minute pace anyway, his body temperature will rise so as to reach the limit of 104°F after only 7 or 8 kilometers. The brain knows this, because it is monitoring feedback, like the rate of the rise in core body temperature, from the outset, as well as the environmental temperature, basing its calculation on previous experience, training, and the race situation.

Obviously, stopping after only 7 kilometers is failure, so rather than simply carrying on blindly until this happens, the brain (or "governor") takes over and reduces muscle activation and hence running pace, as shown in the schematic diagram opposite.

This is not simply a conscious decision. People often dismiss this concept as "obvious," because they know that you have to slow down in the heat. Certainly, you are aware that your pace is slowing, but reduction in muscle activation by the brain seems to precede this conscious awareness and happens despite the fact that the runner is putting forth the same effort. Runners rate their perceived exertion similarly regardless of the temperature, which is crucial, as we'll see shortly.

Our athlete slows down to a 47-minute pace, which means he also produces less heat and is therefore no longer in danger of overheating. When he comes within sight of the finish line, his brain calculates that the danger has passed (there is not enough time to overheat), and thus it allows him to sprint for the line, exhibiting the so-called end spurt.

The most remarkable thing of all is that the brain does much of this unconsciously. The athlete is still trying his hardest, feeling as though he is giving it everything, but the brain knows better. This concept was recently called

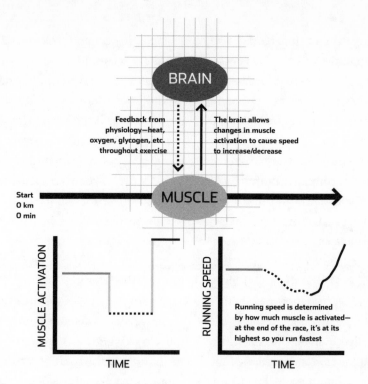

BRAIN

Feedback from
physiology—heat,
oxygen, glycogen, etc.
throughout exercise

The brain allows
changes in muscle
activation to cause speed
to increase/decrease

Start
0 km
0 min

MUSCLE

MUSCLE ACTIVATION

TIME

RUNNING SPEED

Running speed is determined
by how much muscle is activated—
at the end of the race, it's at its
highest so you run fastest

TIME

Anchor points: Where you start, where you finish, and where you are at any given moment in relation to these points

the "anticipatory regulation of exercise," because it all happens in advance of any measurable changes in what are classically thought to be the limiting physiological systems.

The above example applies specifically to exercise in the heat, where the "homeostat" (the physiological parameter that must be defended) is body temperature. However, teleoanticipation is equally adaptable to other situations—exercise at altitude, for example, is probably regulated in much the same way. You will start a 10-K race at 6,000 feet much slower than at sea level, because your brain is aware of the reduced oxygen pressure in the air, thanks to feedback from the body's various systems. Researchers

don't quite know which feedback is most important; it may be the oxygen supply to the brain, or it may be sensed in the lungs, the pulmonary blood vessels, or the muscle. That detail remains to be discovered, but what is certain is that you slow down long before any limit in oxygen delivery develops. Recent research has found that at high altitudes, power output is voluntarily reduced right from the first few seconds of cycling time trials. The classic model of exercise fatigue, which ignores the brain, would predict that power would decrease from its normal low-altitude level during the course of high-altitude time trials because during the trials, the muscle loses its contracting ability later on.

The anticipatory regulation model also applies to fuel availability and glycogen depletion, the limiters. Athletes slow down before they stop, well before they develop a potentially catastrophic level of energy depletion. Research shows that the pacing strategy in athletes who start with less energy is altered almost from the outset. Similarly, during high-intensity exercise such as sprinting, the theory is that a reduction in pH, ATP, and calcium levels plus excessive phosphate and lactate accumulation prevents the muscle from contracting normally, causing fatigue. This is a slightly more complex case, because these metabolites certainly affect muscle function. However, the rapid recovery that is observed after sprinting, plus the fact that a "reserve" exists all the time (you never use all of your muscle fibers, even at maximal effort), suggests that performance is regulated even during short, all-out efforts.

The timing of the changes in running speed is the key aspect relative to heat, altitude, energy restrictions, and high intensity. Fatigue happens *before* failure, in order to prevent it, and this observation represents a departure from the traditional model to explain limits on performance.

The Effect of Motivation, Belief, and Expectation on Running Performance

Now we'll expand the theory to account for how intangibles such as motivation and mental factors affect performance. Classic theory could not account for such factors, as we saw with John Landy. How could a change in mental belief suddenly yield a four-second improvement if the limit existed only in the muscles or heart? We have shown that the limit theory is inadequate and that the brain is in control, regulating performance in response to various signals sent by the body during exercise. What we haven't yet done is explain how motivation, expectation, belief, psychological state, and knowledge of exercise (the so-called soft factors) affect performance.

It's not difficult to see how they might do so, however, if you consider that changes in muscle activation and pacing strategy are the result of how the brain interprets incoming signals during exercise before generating its response. Interpretation of physiological signals opens the door for soft factors such as motivation and belief to influence exercise performance by changing the decision made by the brain in response to the inputs. For example, if you are offered a substantial incentive (money, a medal, fame) to run a PR, chances are you'll tolerate a far greater degree of discomfort than if you ran without incentive or an external motivating factor.

Physiologically, this means that you will be able to maintain a faster running speed, even if the price you pay is a higher body temperature at the end of the race or greater levels of energy depletion. To use a morbid analogy, when scientists have done studies with exercising rats, they have found that if the rats are allowed to stop running whenever they want to, they stop as soon as their body temperature reaches about 104°F. However, if the rats are "motivated" to keep running by means of a small electric shock when they first show signs of slowing down, then they push themselves for much longer and reach much higher body temperatures, around 106°F. When you're chasing your 10-K PR, are you more like the rat that slows down when it begins to approach a high body temperature or more like the "encouraged" rat? It's probably safe to say that all runners are, to some extent, motivated to perform and are therefore more like the shocked rat; some runners approach the absolute limit of exercise performance. These highly motivated individuals are able to run themselves right to the edge of what is possible, accessing just about all available reserves. Ultimately, as mentioned earlier, physiology wins the day—unless there is some pathology that causes fail-safe mechanisms to malfunction, which might include genetic conditions that predispose people to overheating, but little is known about these conditions at present—and you stop before the point of death, the ultimate catastrophe.

Similarly, your attitudes and beliefs toward training and racing have a very significant impact on how you perceive the inevitable discomforts of running. If you decide that the discomfort associated with going out at a pace faster than you've ever done before is acceptable and that the reward outweighs the "punishment," then you are far more likely to tolerate discomfort than if you do not believe this. Emotional state (or affect), levels of motivation, crowd support, and race situations all impact performance in this way. In this regard, the brain is not merely a calculator that spits out an answer to every set of physiological inputs. Instead, it interprets the incoming information in the context of existing emotions, attitudes, and beliefs.

Is it possible that John Landy's ability to cleave 4 seconds off his best time was the result of a seismic shift in his own expectations around performance, courtesy of Roger Bannister's removal of his "brick wall"? We suspect so. Landy had, for three years, been running with the notion of a barrier—the belief that 4 minutes was the target—and his body's ability to break that barrier was constrained by this belief. Once it had been removed, Landy found a new target, and, without the limitation, he was able to reach physiological levels that he had previously found impossible. His degree of muscle activation and hence his fatigue factors, such as muscle acidity, must have been greater in running 3:57.9 than in clocking 4:02, yet he did not tie up at the end of his sub-4 breakthrough. Was this a case of brain over body?

Can We Override the Anticipatory Regulation?

You're probably wondering where this leaves you. Can you overcome regulation by the brain that makes you slow down? The answer is that you can, but only partially. Remember, your brain is doing you a favor, because it is slowing you down before you (a) become prematurely fatigued or (b) hurt yourself by developing heatstroke or some other catastrophic loss of homeostasis. So overriding this mechanism may be harmful—certainly to your performance and possibly to your health. But all is not lost. You are not a slave to your brain, because you can train smart to teach your brain how to be a better orchestra conductor and also learn how to pace yourself better. When the brain decides that you need to slow down and starts activating less muscle, remember that it does so leaving quite a large reserve; this reserve is something that you want to access. You can learn how to access it through diligent and intelligent training. Specifically, training at a range of paces and in a variety of scenarios that prepare your brain-body for the situation you will place it in during the race is a crucial and very effective strategy to break through performance barriers. For a comprehensive discussion of brain training, refer to the book *Brain Training for Runners* (2007), by Matt Fitzgerald.

In terms of pacing yourself, understand the phases of your race and how your physiological systems respond and adapt during the course of the race. It's not ideal to start fast, then slow down dramatically, then speed up again. The ideal pacing strategy is as close to even as possible—the same pace the whole distance, with a slight end spurt in the homestretch. This means that you must train your body to learn this pace and teach your brain that it can allow you to maintain your pace a little longer. Interval training is a great way to do this, and so is running time trials at shorter distances than you plan to race. For example, if you are training for a marathon, go out and run repeats of four kilometers at your race pace, or even slightly faster; be aware that in addition to training your muscles, you are training your brain!

IT'S PART MIND OVER MATTER, PART JUST MATTER

The anticipatory regulation of pacing is not simple psychology. In fact, it's complex physiology. While it has been said that it is mind over matter, the truth is, ultimately, it's still matter, or physiology. This doesn't mean that you should not train your mind, because purely psychological factors such as confidence can be the difference between speeding up and slowing down, between a PR and a disappointment. By doing regular interval training, you'll not only learn how to think when you run and how to override your desire to stop, but also teach your brain and your body how to run at your goal pace. And that equals personal-best performances.

Chapter 12

It's All about Style

Running is a basic activity. If you want to get technical, take up ballet or golf, where you practice for hours in an attempt to perfect very specific movements. Or join a karate studio, where an instructor will teach you *how* to perform that activity. Even in swimming, coaches apply an expert eye and make adjustments to arm movement, body position, use of the legs, and so on. But running? That's inherent. We just do it. Right?

Not necessarily. Coaches and athletes have long recognized that small changes to running form, such as adjustments to arm and head position, shoulder relaxation, the "lean" of your body, and your stride characteristics (stride length and rate) may affect running performance. We all marvel at the beautifully fluid and relaxed running style of the East African runners, often remarking how smooth and comfortable they look. But pinpointing precisely what it is that creates this impression is not quite so simple—it is even beyond the capabilities of science, which has studied running technique (a vast and complex term that encompasses, quite literally, everything from head to toe), concluding that variations in body proportion and size explain most of the differences in running technique.

According to this notion, there cannot be a "one size fits all" technique. Rather, each individual has an optimal technique that is as unique to him or her as a fingerprint. This unique quality is clear when you watch any world-class marathon race. You can compare the smooth, natural style of Martin Lel to the compact elasticity of Haile Gebrselassie and contrast this with the stocky, punchy style of Olympic champion Sammy Wanjiru and the seemingly tense and wasteful head movements and high arm carry of Paula Radcliffe. It's difficult to suggest that any of these world-class runners should change his or her technique to run faster—there is a good chance it would do more harm than good.

So, rather than attempt to simplify this impossibly large topic to the running equivalent of a technical manual, coaches and athletes have tended to adopt a "seven habits of highly effective runners" approach, in which they develop golden rules, or principles, that should be obeyed within a necessarily flexible framework. These principles, which we'll cover in this chapter, usually pertain to the position of the head, shoulders, arms, and hips, as well as stride length and, perhaps most commonly, the landing of the foot.

However, a growing number of running technique advocates have emerged, and the skill of running has been sold like never before. Numerous books, DVDs, and video packages are touted as holding the secret to unlocking your speed and reaching your potential, all while staying injury-free. These methods are different from the traditional approach to running technique, because they don't simply suggest a few things that should be modified on a case-by-case basis; they actually advocate that your current running technique is flawed and that you need a major technique overhaul, relearning how to run correctly and then practicing a set of prescribed exercises, just as you would in a sport such as golf.

Is "Natural" Wrong? Do We Run Incorrectly?

Implicit in this approach is the notion that your natural running technique is incorrect. In other words, your running style is broken, so now fix it! The concept that we might run "incorrectly" is not too radical when you compare running with other sports activities. No one picks up a tennis racket and just happens to learn the perfect forehand. Players must be coached, or else they learn bad habits and technique. But we tend to think of running a bit differently. We progress from crawling to walking and then running and think of it as innate. But the running technique advocates suggest that many, if not most, of us learn this ability incorrectly (or nonoptimally, to use a gentler word).

One of the most widely practiced running technique offerings is the Pose running technique. If you spend some time on the Pose Tech Web site, you'll find that it addresses the "natural style" question with a lengthy explanation. The argument is that we erroneously accept that natural is best. Here's a quote from the Pose site: "So, no matter how you run, it's ok [sic]. If you try to apply this 'logic' to any other human activity such as swimming, tennis, dancing, driving a car and so on, it would sound totally strange, but not so for running."

The point of the essay is that we've missed something because we perceive running to be a basic task that anyone can perform. It is a compelling argument, given credence by the fact that injury rates are the same today as they were 30 years ago, despite improved coaching, better medical care, and better running shoes. Therefore, according to supporters of technique philosophies such as Pose and Chi running, our running technique must be bad. This observation is a key selling point for the systematic teaching of specific running technique systems.

What do we make of this argument? Is there any reason to believe it's true? Again, science is not particularly helpful on this matter, so it remains mainly a philosophical argument for now. But a commonsense critical evaluation of the argument suggests that it probably overreaches.

THE INJURY CONFOUNDER

To begin with, the often-cited injury statistic is a little misleading, because the typical runner of today is not the typical runner of 30 years ago. Thirty years ago, runners were "born to run"—mass events were uncommon, the running industry had not yet exploded, and most runners were *competitive* runners: small, lightweight, and probably exhibiting similar biomechanics (in terms of anthropometrical measurements: leg length, skeletal structure, and so on). Today, anyone can run (and does!), from the 100-pound elite superstar of 30 years ago to the 250-pound weekend warrior. The inclusiveness of running, as evidenced by the sport's phenomenal growth

over the past few decades, is a wonderful thing. But it also provides an alternative explanation for why people get injured. A preponderance of today's noncompetitive runners, who don't share the physical condition or biomechanical traits of the elite, are likely to become injured with even the tiniest error in training, regardless of how good their running technique is.

To consider some hypothetical numbers, 30 years ago perhaps 1 million people were running, and 500,000 got injured. Today, 10 million people are running, and 5 million get injured. One possible interpretation of these figures is that because the prevalence of injury is the same (50 percent) despite better shoes and knowledge, we must run incorrectly. This is what the Pose and Chi creators suggest. The alternative view is that today, 4.5 million more people are running without injury than 30 years ago! Sure, 4.5 million more people are injured, too, but given that most of these people probably do not have the ideal running build for running, their presence in the sample compromises its integrity as an apples-to-apples comparison. In this case, the *same* actually represents a pretty solid improvement.

RUNNING TECHNIQUE: IS RUNNING THE SAME AS A TENNIS SWING?

Returning to the fundamental issue of whether running should be taught as a skill, like swimming, dancing, and golf, there is an even more philosophical debate. You don't, for example, have to teach children how to walk. They just do it, learning from trial and error how to distribute their balance. They fall backward, they overbalance, they stand in place, but eventually they get it right.

You don't even have to teach a person how to ride a bike—all you do is facilitate the learning opportunity, and the person falls over until eventually he figures out how to distribute his weight correctly! Once learned, the movement is natural. At this point you might ask, "Where do you draw the line between what is learned naturally and what is taught technically?" And that is the million-dollar question.

Running technique philosophies such Pose and Chi running challenge the widely held perception that each person naturally figures out how to run more or less optimally for his or her body. But if the Pose and Chi methods are correct and it is indeed incorrect running technique that is the primary cause of running injuries, the next important question to ask is why don't we automatically run in the most efficient way possible? Evolutionary biologists believe that humans learned to run for survival; therefore would we not have developed an effective running technique that maximized our capacity for flight and pursuit? Humans used to run for their very lives—either toward the food they craved or away from becoming it! In this regard, running is different from tennis. No one ever compromised his survival because he couldn't hit a topspin forehand! But in prehistoric times, if you ran badly and developed stress fractures or runner's knee, your poor technique would have had serious consequences.

In recent years, some of the best scientific papers on running have come from anthropologists and sports scientists in the United States looking at how humans are adapted to run—specifically, at how our skeleton, tendons, and thermoregulatory system differ from those of our primate cousins. The point is that running is not an arbitrary skill like swinging a golf club or hitting a forehand down the line in tennis. It's something that lies on our developmental path as children, a learned progression after crawling and walking. Quite why we'd learn it incorrectly is difficult to explain. One might counter this line of questioning by pointing out that only a small minority of humans have any real talent for distance running—an undeniable fact that makes the argument that we are evolved for distance running ability appear rather weak. After all, every cheetah is a great sprinter, while only the tiniest fraction of humans have a gift for endurance running. So perhaps this ability was only ever needed by a small group of specialists throughout human evolution; in fact most of us are *not* highly evolved for distance running (although compared with other primates, even the least gifted runners among us are superstars). But even with this qualification, it seems unlikely that poor technique, independent of body structure, is what holds back the weaker human runners—think instead of cardiovascular capacity, metabolic system limitations, muscle types, and neurological factors that combine to separate the world-class runners from the everyday joggers.

The most common explanation for the high injury rate in running put forward by today's technique advocates is that the running shoe has driven the emergence of incorrect technique, because the added cushioning allows you to make nonoptimal changes in how your feet land during running. Specifically, you can, thanks to air bubbles, gel pads, and EVA cushioning, land on your heel rather than your forefoot. The supposedly perfect running technique of the Kenyans is attributed to the fact that they don't run in shoes for much of their early lives. This controversial issue will be touched on later—and it is a provocative one.

Proponents of the more traditional view of running technique counter that this argument is meaningless, because it suggests that the only way to run correctly is to throw away your shoes and run barefoot—a surefire way to get injured quickly. But few if any "new-school" technique advocates tell runners to throw away their shoes. Instead, most advocate the use of lighter, lower-profile shoes that facilitate a midfoot landing, and they argue that it is possible to override the natural ten-dency to heel-strike in shoes with a conscious effort. And indeed there are many thousands of runners who profess to have changed their footstrike pattern successfully without going barefoot.

Yet can we really be certain that this change is beneficial? After all, if your body naturally shifts from a heel-striking to a midfoot-striking running style for self-protection when switching from shod to barefoot running, might it not also be the case that switching from a forefoot-striking to a heel-striking running style when putting on shoes is also protective? Quite why the body would protect you by shifting to a forefoot landing when barefoot but not the other way around has never been explained. We'll pick this issue up when we discuss forefoot versus heel striking later in this chapter.

Taking an even broader view, it's difficult to fathom how millions of people would collectively, yet independently, get their technique so wrong. It's not as though everyone is being fed the same message. Surely it would not have taken until the 1990s for "ideal" technique to be discovered and packaged for those misguided runners?

Also, the notion that millions of people, with different body shapes and sizes and leg lengths and centers of gravity and joint angles, could fit into one single pattern or technique is also difficult to accept. Rather, the passage of time would filter out any flaws for each person.

That said, we're not dismissing the importance of running technique, because it's an area with little concrete evidence but plenty of experience and potential benefit for you as a runner. What we do think untenable is the possibility that wholesale changes, advocated by the packaged running technique offerings, hold the answer to faster and safer running. It's not to say that Pose, Chi, or any of the other running techniques are completely flawed, because they do make some pretty good fundamental arguments. But we're interested in *your* running, and therefore we need to understand what the truly universal principles of effective running technique are and how they might be applied to you specifically, rather than to everyone including you. The next step, then, is to consider the elements of running technique.

Running Technique: Earning Style Points

An entire book could be written about the basics of running technique, but that's certainly not our objective here. So we begin with the initial disclaimer that the topic is simply too vast and complex to summarize fully. When discussing the perfect running technique, the temptation is to copy the example of the runners who you think embody "perfection." You would think that you could do a lot worse than modeling yourself on a world record holder or an Olympic champion!

This approach suffers from a practical problem: Which aspects you can or should copy are not as obvious as you might think. Obviously, only a fool would suggest that you copy idiosyncrasies such as Paula Radcliffe's unique rolling head motion. Nor would anyone recommend that every runner emulate technique characteristics that only a minority of elite runners exhibit, such as Gebrselassie's widely perceived forefoot landing style. Rather, the only characteristics of elite running technique that should be copied are those that truly define the elites as a group and seem practically duplicable by non-elite runners. Very few such characteristics have been identified, however.

Yet there are some. For example, research has shown that faster runners make ground contact with a stiffer, tenser leg than slower runners. A stiffer leg on landing is able to capture more "free energy" from ground impact forces and return it into the ground to propel forward motion. Leg stiffness is achieved by preactivation of the leg muscles just before the foot lands. It seems reasonable that any runner, regardless of body structure, could practice preactivating their leg muscles more when running and perhaps thereby gain a little efficiency.

Whether preactivation for greater leg stiffness truly represents a universal principle of good running technique is unknown, however, because like most other proposed principles, it has been neither fully validated nor refuted by science. This is because the study required to examine optimal technique is virtually impossible to perform. There are simply too many variables to control, thanks to the unique individual attributes that apparently produce technique differences. A specific change in technique (for example, having runners change stride length) might produce changes in certain physiological measurements (such as heart rate, VO$_2$ max, and so on), but that doesn't necessarily translate into better performance. And finally, any interference with technique by a scientist is guaranteed to worsen it, at least initially, because it takes a runner time to adjust to even a potentially beneficial change. So no study is able to tell you that doing A is better than doing B, because directly measuring and comparing cause and effect is impossible. Therefore, we have to adopt a pragmatic, theoretical view of running technique.

HEAD AND SHOULDERS: SOURCES OF RELAXATION

The head and shoulders tell the body what "mood" to be in. Tension often originates in the head, face, and shoulders. Whenever athletes tie up or get tense, the first place it's evident is in the neck and shoulders. You will no doubt have seen this on television when elite athletes race down the home straight of Olympic finals. The corollary to this point is that the head and shoulders determine the degree of relaxation when running, and just

about anything you can do to relax when running is beneficial, because relaxation equals energy conservation. There are, as with most things, exceptions to this "rule." Paula Radcliffe has been used as an example twice in this chapter, thanks to her habit of rolling her head from side to side, particularly toward the latter stages of a race (including her world record 2:15 marathon). We would suggest that her excessive head movement, which many have suggested is a detrimental factor, is in fact a *source* of relaxation. That is, movement doesn't imply tension, and perhaps if Radcliffe forced a steady head position, she'd tighten up where it counts—in the trunk and legs.

To relax from the top down, start with your mouth, jaw, neck, and shoulders. Many athletes, particularly as novices, suffer from cramping and pain in the shoulders—that's nothing more than tension. Drop your arms; don't hunch your shoulders. Just let your arms hang loosely, and the pain usually goes away. The best time to practice this conscious "top-down" relaxation is during speed sessions, when you are most likely to tense up. As with many skills, relaxing obeys the adage "Practice makes perfect."

ARMS: THE JOCKEY

The arms are the "jockey" to the body and legs, which are the "horse." In long-distance running, the arms play a far less important role than in sprints, where arm movement provides a counterbalance to the torque and forces being applied to the trunk by the legs as they swing through. This is also the role of the arms during distance running, but it's far less critical. Perhaps the two biggest factors to think of here are fatigue and tension. Fatigue tends to become a problem in shorter, higher-intensity running, when the arms are used more. The only way to address this issue is to get your arms used to short, fast efforts, which will increase their fatigue resistance. There are no shortcuts.

Tension is a more immediately rectifiable problem. If the arms become tense, that tension once again filters to the rest of the body. The hands in particular are important—clenched fists and tight, rigid wrists are signs of tension, so try to consciously relax these areas, remembering also that tension in the arms is often the result of tension in the shoulders, neck, and face, as explained.

Excessive arm movement is discouraged, because it increases the energy cost of running. As we saw when discussing running economy in Chapter 5, distance running is about getting more mileage per milliliter, and wasting energy on arm movement is not a helpful strategy in the long run (literally). If you're worried that your arms are moving excessively, then they probably are, because as we've said, the arms follow the pattern dictated by the legs. Only when you begin working very hard—during speedwork, in shorter races, and at the end of races—does arm

movement begin to contribute significantly to running faster.

The optimal position of the arms is up for debate. Generally, an elbow angle between 80 and 100 degrees is natural, but there are exceptions. Chinese runner Junxia Wang runs like a soldier, with virtually straight arms. This may not be the most effective way to run, but I suspect that anything else she tried would be unsuccessful.

A similar principle holds for arm swing. Some athletes swing their arms across their body; others advocate a much straighter arm swing. You may have been told that your hands should not cross the midline of your body, for example. In other words, don't let your right hand come across to the left half of your body. Again, that's a dogmatic guideline that simply doesn't fit with what is observed in runners, and it depends on the person. Kenenisa Bekele has not heard this advice, for example (or if he did, he ignored it). Perhaps the most important guideline for arm carry and swing is that you don't "suffocate" yourself by carrying your arms too tightly. The buzzword, once again, is *relaxation*.

HIPS: THE CENTER OF MASS AND THE SOURCE OF FORWARD MOVEMENT

The hips are crucially important because they determine, to a large extent, where the center of mass is during running. This is where the Pose Method is conceptually strong and has used biomechanical principles correctly. If your foot were to land well in front of your center of mass, you would decelerate. Think of a long jumper, who virtually comes to a halt as a result of throwing his legs out in front of his hips. Ideally, the hips should be as high and as far forward as possible, within reason. In other words, break at the hips as though you are going to sit down. The best way to feel this breaking effect is to drop your hips slightly next time you are running downhill. Because you're on a descent, your center of mass will go backward, and you'll feel an immediate loss of momentum.

In contrast, if you want to speed up on a downhill, simply lean forward—not at the shoulders, but by tilting your whole body forward just a little. Think of trying to reach up to get a jar off the top shelf of a cupboard—you have to stretch upward *and* lean forward. That's what you need to do with your hips if you want to accelerate during running, even on level ground.

This is not easy for runners who don't do it naturally. It requires strong core muscles. Do some Pilates or gym training to strengthen these muscles to make it easier for you to lift your hips and lean forward for more speed.

One of the most common running technique mistakes is to lean forward at the shoulders. The problem is that it pushes your hips backward. This is most noticeable up hills, where the temptation is to hunch forward. Not only does hunching hinder breathing,

but it actually destroys your efficiency. Instead, concentrate on leaning from the ankles, so that your hips are forward. It sometimes even helps to pull your shoulders back, as though you are standing in a soldier's upright, "at-attention" position.

THE KNEES AND STRIDE CHARACTERISTICS

"Drive your knees forward! Come on, pick the knees up!" That's the universal cry of coaches who want athletes to speed up. The problem is that driving forward with the knees is actually counterproductive. It usually results in overstriding, artificially increasing stride length by "bounding," because this is the only way a tired athlete can obey the instruction. The energy cost of bounding is enormous, consuming substantially more energy than normal running. Also, when you overstride, your foot lands way out in front of your center of mass. This causes braking and deceleration, which then means you have to work even harder to speed up or maintain a speed. So the instruction to lift the knees is probably not a good one.

Instead of trying to lift your knees, think about lifting your feet off the ground. This is another element that the Pose technique advocates, and it's certainly correct in principle. Far from being revolutionary, however, it's common sense and is seen in the running style of most elite runners, who perform a "heel flick" at the top of the stride. It's a result of the realization that being light on the feet is a crucial characteristic of good running technique.

From a practical point of view, it's important not to overload your mind with all sorts of instructions, lest running become a mental endurance test as much as a physical one. But the simple concept of pulling your foot up underneath you is easy to achieve and makes a difference. Try to imagine that you are running on eggshells or thin ice and that you need to flick the ground very lightly, and you'll start to teach your brain to activate the right muscles more effectively.

A natural consequence of running "lightly" is reduced contact time on the ground, and this will mean that your stride rate (also called cadence) will increase. Other things remaining equal (stride length, in particular), you'll speed up significantly as a result. For example, at the end of your next race, notice that your finishing burst is the result of an increase in both stride length and stride rate. You can learn the faster stride rate through practice in training sessions. Of course, your heart and lungs will not agree with your newly learned supercharged running technique, so you have to take care to train the other systems to match this mechanical improvement. This is why structured sessions in which you focus on both a lighter landing and deliberate change in muscle activation are recommended. Don't simply head out and force your cadence higher during your normal six-mile loop. Our advice is to build short sections of stride-rate training into your sessions, particularly speedwork sets, in which you can recover between intervals. For example, after completing a one-mile easy jogging warmup, run four to six "strides" of 100 yards at a moderately fast pace, concentrating on running lightly with fast turnover. Rest for 30 seconds between strides. After completing your strides, move into the main body of your speed workout.

When they consciously increase stride rate, runners tend to unconsciously decrease their stride length. This is natural, and one of the few Pose running studies found exactly this result. But you don't have to practice Pose running to achieve the same result. It will happen regardless of how you achieve the faster stride rate, including following our suggestion of building in shorter periods of focused "lighter" running in your speed workouts. It's important, however, that you do not force yourself into a stride rate that is, say, 10 percent higher than your normal rate. For example, you currently take 85 strides a minute, but Haile Gebrselassie takes 95, so you force a 10-stride-per-minute increase. Such a drastic change would almost certainly come at the cost of reduced economy. Many runners are preoccupied with stride rate and force themselves into a rate that they believe to be optimal by counting strides, often using music to dictate the tempo. This is more likely to be detrimental to your running; you'd be better off focusing on one change—a lighter landing courtesy of the activation of the hamstring muscles—and letting stride rate take care of itself.

THE FEET: THE MOST IMPORTANT (AND CONTROVERSIAL) OF ALL

Perhaps the most heavily discussed technique aspect of all is the footstrike. Runners have become increasingly preoccupied with how and where the foot strikes the ground during running. Take for example the following information given to beginning runners as part of a package that includes advice on running technique:

> *Do not allow your heel to strike the ground first; this causes a jolt up your leg and reduces the efficiency of your leg joints. If you keep your ankle soft your foot should land anywhere between the ball and the middle of your sole. This allows for a "springier" action and gets a better push up from the floor.*

The basic message is that heel striking is inefficient and causes injury. Midfoot or forefoot striking is the desired landing style. This dogma is certainly open to debate. In fact, even the three authors of this book do not agree. On this matter, Ross and Jonathan favor the view that heel striking is probably best for most runners who land this way naturally, while Matt favors the new-school view that most heel-strikers can and should train them-selves to at least become less-pronounced heel-strikers, if not midfoot-strikers. This is not necessarily a disagreement about the merits of the different footstrike patterns, for these are not really known, but is more a function of the fact that changing the footstrike carries with it certain risks (if done improperly) that are not offset by the potential (and unknown) benefits.

With regard to the risk, most runners respond to advice such as that we quoted above by focusing only on the landing point, completely missing the key point about "keeping the ankle soft" (another example of relaxation—our buzzword). They then become preoccupied with whether they are landing on the heel, the midfoot, or the forefoot. This is a recipe for injury, because the mental concern about landing causes excessive tension in the wrong muscles and, with it, muscle tissue strain.

If you ever watch runners trying to follow this advice on their own, you will see that almost all of them deliberately contract their calves to put their ankle joints into what we call plantar flexion (pointing the toes away from the body) before they land. As a result, they land on the forefoot, but the poor calf muscle bears the brunt of the body weight while it is contracted. Not surprisingly, calf muscle injuries are pretty common in people who try to implement this advice.

New-schoolers counter that this common problem is easily avoided if the runner who is interested in changing his or her footstrike pattern is properly guided. They contend that the previously discussed technique error of overstriding is inextricably linked to that of heel striking, such that the latter error is automatically corrected when the error of overstriding is properly addressed. To see how overstriding and heel striking are linked, perform the following simple experiment: In a standing position, flex the hip and knee of one leg so that your foot rises away from the floor directly in line with your body. Now put your foot back down. How does it land? On the midfoot. Now take a step forward with the same leg. How does the foot land? Heel first.

So the argument is that anyone who grants that the foot should land under the body during running, rather than out ahead of it, should also grant that the foot should land flat, not heel first. In any case, in training yourself to touch your foot down beneath your hips, you are very likely to become a less-pronounced heel-striker, or even a true midfoot-striker, whether you intend to or not. If you can do this successfully, then you'll also avoid the potentially dangerous temptation of "reaching" for the landing with your toe pointed down, and this is the key to getting the change right.

THE FOOTSTRIKE DEBATE: HEEL VERSUS FOREFOOT

As you can see, footstrike patterns represent a controversial point in our technique discussion. The debate has been stoked by the discussion of shod versus barefoot running and especially by the argument that the only reason we land on the heel is because shoe cushioning gives us license to do so. Landing on the midfoot is the natural, barefoot way and must therefore be better. As mentioned, old-schoolers point out that this notion ignores the fact that the shift to heel striking in shoes may be as much an adaptation to optimize running as the shift to midfoot landing when the shoes come off. The argument has only ever been presented one way. While there is no question that the built-up, elevated heel of shoes promotes heel striking, no one has established a greater risk of injury when people run this way.

What about the argument that midfoot striking is more economical and facilitates greater speed than heel striking? This argument has received some scientific attention, but as you will soon see, the attention has brought us no closer to an answer.

WHAT DO THE ELITES DO? FOOTSTRIKE PATTERNS IN ELITE ATHLETES

An interesting and relevant study on footstrike patterns emerged out of Japan recently. Elite athletes running the 2004 Sapporo International Half Marathon were studied using high-speed cameras to capture their feet at the 15-kilometer mark. The researchers from Ryukoku University managed to observe

248 men and 35 women and characterized them as either heel-strikers, midfoot-strikers, or forefoot-strikers. They also measured ground contact time at the 15-kilometer point.

The main findings:

→ The vast majority (75 percent) of elite runners landed on the heel.

→ About one in four runners (24 percent) landed on the midfoot.

→ Only four out of 283 runners landed on the forefoot.

This breakdown is shown graphically below.

Given this result, one is tempted to say that the landing of the foot has no bearing on running performance.

However, there are two reasons why this conclusion might be too hasty. First, as some commentators on this study have pointed out, all heel-strikers are not equal. Distributing the full spectrum of footstriking patterns among just three categories—heel-strikers, midfoot-strikers, and forefoot-strikers—is a bit like classifying every human stature as either short, medium, or tall. Suppose we decided that any adult standing less than 5'2" was short, that any adult standing between 5'3" and 5'10" was medium in height, and that

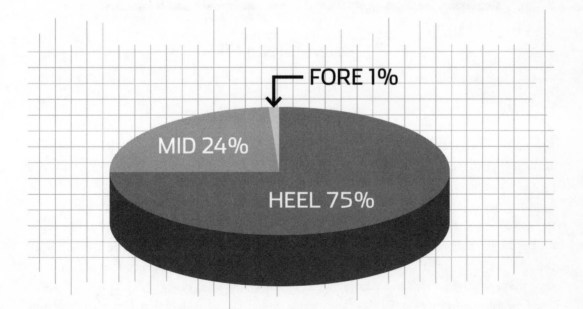

FORE 1%

MID 24%

HEEL 75%

Footstrike pattern and ground contact for elite athletes

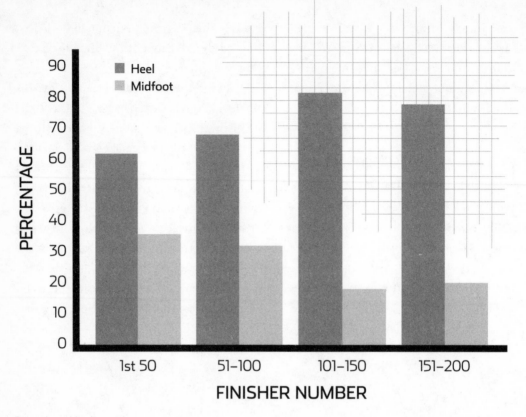

Footstrike and finisher number

anyone who stood 5'11" or taller was tall. According to this classification, a 5'10" person and another at 5'11" would be in two completely different height categories despite the fact that they stand nearly eye-to-eye.

Similarly, there are infinite gradations in footstrike points between the very back of the heel and the very front of the forefoot, such that the three categories actually blend. And it is all but certain that the elite runners who were classified as heel-strikers in the Ryukoku University study were not heel-strikers in the same way that the average model/jogger pictured in a stock photograph used in commercial advertising—with his forward leg reaching ridiculously far in front of his body and his ankle cocked back at a painfully acute angle, bracing for impact—is a heel-striker. Indeed, the study under discussion shows sample images of foot landings from each category, and the example of heel striking is barely distinguishable from that of midfoot striking.

Second, when the researchers divided the

finishers into groups of 50 based on their finishing order, they saw a distinct correlation between speed and footstrike pattern. There was a higher percentage of heel-strikers in the first 50 runners than in the second, between the second and the third, and so on. The graph opposite shows this relationship between heel-strikers and midfoot-strikers.

At first glance, the conclusion drawn from this graph could be that if you want to be a faster runner, finishing higher up in the overall ranking, then you should be a midfoot-striker, not a heel-striker. That's how many people interpreted the finding. And this may well be true. There is, however, another possible reason it looks like it does: Perhaps it's simply a function of running faster.

Speed and Footstrike

As you increase your running speed, you naturally shift your contact point with the ground farther forward. The average speed, incidentally, of the first 50 runners in the Ryukoku study was 3:03 per kilometer. The second group of 50 runners averaged 3:10 per kilometer. Hardly a big difference, but given the range (the 50th runner was at least a minute behind the first runner at the finish line), it is possible that all this finding shows is the effect of running speed on footstrike.

To get a personal feel for the relationship between speed and footstrike patterns, try the following experiment: Go down to your local track and sprint 100 meters, noting how you land. Chances are you'll be landing on your forefeet, possibly even your toes, the whole way. Because you are running faster, you shift your landing toward the forefoot.

During your sprint, you'll probably cover 100 meters in 14 seconds, which puts you only 1 second ahead of the pace that a Bekele or a Gebrselassie sustains in a 5000-meter race, so is it any wonder they are midfoot-strikers on the track? They're running as fast as most of us sprint! The point is that if you ran their speed, you'd probably be a midfoot-striker too!

That said, if you have ever had the experience of watching elite runners warm up for a race, you might have noticed that most of them remain very mild heel-strikers or midfoot-strikers even at the slowest speeds. While everyone gets on their toes to sprint (it's a quantum shift, like that which occurs between walking and running at much slower speeds), most runners maintain a fairly consistent footstrike pattern at submaximal speeds. Taken to its extreme, the argument that footstrike pattern is dependent on speed implies that every runner lands on the same spot on the foot at any given speed, and this is obviously not the case. It also does not explain why all barefoot runners are midfoot- or forefoot-strikers at all speeds.

At any rate, this study does not allow you to differentiate between three possibilities:

1. Faster runners are midfoot-strikers (could be coincidence or some other cause).

2. Midfoot-strikers are faster runners (and therefore we should all change our running style and land on the middle part of the foot).

3. All runners would eventually be midfoot-strikers if they ran fast enough.

Old-schoolers see possibility 3 as the most likely. They ask, why should you try to run with the same footstrike as the fastest elite when you are running perhaps three minutes per kilometer slower than they are? It just makes no sense to copy the elite runner's footstrike when you are running so much slower—the only result of this imitation is likely to be injury.

New-school technique advocates favor possibility 2. They argue that a midfoot strike facilitates faster running, that midfoot-strikers are midfoot-strikers at any speed (except when sprinting, when we all suddenly become forefoot-strikers), and that any runner can become a midfoot-striker, or at least a less-pronounced heel-striker. In fact, if you are able to overcome overstriding, you will "correct" your landing style automatically.

Conclusion

Discussions of running technique tend to inspire some rather sensitive responses in the running community—right up there with religion and political affiliation! This is a sign of just how personal running technique is and that every runner tends to take ownership of perhaps the only thing he or she can. We've tried to cover this enormous topic in as much detail as possible without making what we believe to be the common mistake of being dogmatic or narrow-minded in how we interpret running technique.

The running community has long been preoccupied with running technique, and often with good reason. But the newer trend toward making wholesale changes in technique, based on the assumption that we tend to run incorrectly if left to our own devices, is a more radical approach, one the author's of this book don't advocate (although one of us sees a wider scope for technique training than the other two). In our opinion, then, running is an activity that is:

→ First learned naturally, then . . .

→ Refined through practice, and then . . .

→ Can be subtly changed through instruction on a case-by-case basis.

When we write that running is a natural activity, bear in mind that "natural" does not mean "optimal." So while nearly everyone can run, not everyone who can run runs *well*. The key question is whether one can (or should) be instructed in a comprehensive, one-size-fits-all technique. That is, after all, what both Pose and Chi running offer. Our position is to avoid such approaches, but that does not necessarily mean there are not some sound principles and concepts in those running techniques that runners can cherry-pick and benefit from adopting.

Finally, bear in mind that technique, if we define it as a skill, can be improved in much the same way as any other skill—through practice. Just as a tennis player has to hit many balls and a golfer spends hours on the range, so, too, running properly requires practice. Every runner's stride improves automatically in subtle ways as he or she becomes fitter. In fact, such improvement is a big part of what getting fitter really is. Of course, there is a chance that people will learn or develop bad habits. And this is where the instruction in and application of certain technical drills can make a difference. An informed coach, a knowledgeable observer, or even an intuitive runner can adapt and modify technique so that it conforms with a better theoretical model of running.

There almost certainly is a better way to run, but there certainly is *not* only one correct way to run. So don't place yourself in the same box that the most dogmatic technique advocates do. Work with what you have, make intelligent choices, be patient, and seek to constantly improve but never radically redefine your running. And remember to relax!

Chapter 13

The Joy of Running

Running has turned many a life around. There are countless happy tales of men and women who reclaimed their minds and lives in one way or another through running. Let's consider a single case study that is unique in its particulars but wonderfully typical in its general contours. Susan, 34, is a clinical psychologist who lives in the Los Angeles area. She describes herself as "hungry for life now." But as her qualifying use of the word "now" suggests, it wasn't always that way.

As Susan remembers it, she "hid from life" from the time she was a small girl until she experienced a kind of rebirth at age 25, when she became a runner. Her hiding took two forms: an almost constant state of melancholy that she concealed from herself and the world through a variety of diversionary tactics, which were mostly unhealthy; and a classic "mortification of the flesh"—that is, a pathological denial of her body's needs.

It was the usual suspect, family dysfunction, that caused Susan to experience these symptoms. It could have been worse. She describes her parents, who were and are still together, as basically good people. Her father, a responsible and driven man, made a solid living as a salesman for a large manufacturer of business machines. Her mother, a full-time homemaker, was loving and attentive. And she was the second of four bright, gifted, and beautiful children.

However, there were problems. The anxious and high-strung personalities of both of Susan's parents created a household atmosphere of constant tension. Everyone in the family was expected to excel in all undertakings, and for the most part everyone did so, which only intensified their anxiety. Susan's father could not express his feelings well and had no idea how to relate to his daughter, while her mother lived so vicariously through her only female child that it was "totally suffocating," Susan says. Also, her older brother bullied her mercilessly in a childish effort to redirect the anxiety he absorbed from the family culture.

If Susan had suffered nothing worse, the psychological problems she brought into adulthood probably would have been less severe. But Susan was also sexually molested by a close relative outside her nuclear family, and worse, her nuclear family refused to acknowledge it when Susan courageously blew the whistle, and thereafter.

One partial solution Susan found for the unhappiness she felt was literal escape. "I was definitely much happier when I was away from the house. So from a very early age I learned how to go and make myself a kid at other people's homes," she says. From this strategy developed the gregariousness that became the most effective means of concealing her unhappiness from herself and others. "I never would have considered myself to be depressed," she explains, "although now that I'm a professional, I can look back and say, 'Wow, there was a lot of sadness there'—probably a constant, low-grade depression. I could swing out of it, though. Fortunately, because I was very popular, there were a lot of fun things that happened and some good times."

A far less healthy way of dealing with the unhappiness was Susan's choice to live outside her body as much as possible. For example, this predisposition, coupled with the attention she received on account of being pretty and sweet-natured, inspired her to begin her first "diet" at age 9—and to remain on it straight through to her early adulthood, when it became a bona fide eating disorder. "It was the classic 'I'm not eating' diet," she says. "When I was 15, I would eat an apple and a Snickers bar for lunch. I was totally out of touch with any nutritional needs of the body."

Disembodied as she was, Susan was not likely to have become an athlete as a child, and in the context of her family, it was out of the question. This was because running became the primary means by which the males of Susan's family expressed their "achievement complex." Susan's father ran every single morning, and he completed a marathon when she was about 10 years old. Inspired by their father, Susan's younger brothers ran a marathon—26.2 miles—at ages 8 and 9, while Mike, the eldest, did the same at age 14. And not only did the three brothers complete marathons, but they were also terrific runners. In fact, Mike went on to actually *win* marathons and triathlons. Susan felt totally shut out of all this, and she *was* shut out. "I wanted to do what they did," she says, "because it looked like fun, so I would try things, but everything I did, Mike was threatened by, so he would humiliate me, which spoiled it. So I learned not to try. I just decided that those things were not for me."

Becoming an adult is difficult for almost everyone, but it is especially hard for those who have not healed the wounds of their childhood. This was the case for Susan, who in college went from denying her body to abusing it by essentially starving herself, smoking cigarettes, drinking far too much alcohol, and using other drugs, ranging from marijuana to cocaine and amphetamines. Fortunately, this self-destructive phase did not last long; unfortunately, it did not end in a solution to the underlying problem. "That was not the person I envisioned myself to be and not the person I wanted to be," Susan says of her party animal self. "When I really felt it getting out of control, I was able to stop. However, after one stops such things, there's this sort of elated period that follows, and then it's just depression, because the drugs were masking all of the sadness that was there."

A few years later, Susan received an invitation from a longtime friend to begin jogging with her. Susan was then working full-time and studying for her master's degree. She was still unhappy but actively in search of healing. When she accepted her friend's invitation, she did so with a modest degree of hope and enthusiasm. She hoped that she would enjoy it and experience some of the benefits it had given her father and three brothers, but she did not expect it to precipitate a complete "rebirth," as she describes it. However, that's precisely what it did.

"We started running together at a very slow pace, and something just shifted in me," she recalls. "I don't even know if I could have defined what was happening at the time. I just felt happier and more powerful. I began to feel like I could do anything. The depression that I had felt was totally replaced with joy. That was the first step, and it became a catalyst for so many big changes."

The more Susan progressed in her running, the further she progressed in her personal transformation. Step by step, she worked her way up to longer and longer runs and eventually began to participate in road races: An initial five-miler was followed by a half-marathon, then a marathon, then another, and another, and so on. "Being able to run three miles, I just wanted to slap myself a high five!" she says. "And everything I did beyond that—my first run alone, my first race—made me feel so good and so proud of myself. By the time I did the half-marathon, it was so much a part of my self-concept. I just knew that it was something I would do forever."

There were other benefits. The more she got into running, the more Susan's stress levels decreased. She began to sleep better and to experience far more energy in her waking hours. As a result, she was able to get a much better handle on her challenging schedule and find greater success and enjoyment in the pursuit of her professional degree. Today, her days remain very long and crammed with activity, and she wouldn't have it any other way.

Even more profound was the improvement in her sense of personal ability. One of her favorite stories concretizes the link between running and this welcome change. Says Susan, "I remember having a moment after running a marathon when I was driving to work and my car got a flat tire. I was on a freeway overpass, so it was a dangerous place, and I had never changed a tire in my life. I said, 'You know what? You've just run a marathon; I'm pretty sure you can handle this tire thing.' I've used that as a metaphor for so many things in my life. I don't necessarily have that same dialogue with myself any longer, but that power and that confidence are still with me. I am an extremely confident person now. I can walk into just about any situation and feel like I can handle it.

"I do some of my work in a prison," she continues. "I work with some pretty disturbed people, and nothing freaks me out. I've been in situations where chairs are flying, and I'm a small woman, but I will come into the room and yell, 'Knock it off!'—and they do. And I can trace it all back to the running."

Susan made progress in the interpersonal dimension, as well. As she discovered herself, she found the perspective and the strength she needed to improve important relationships—and end them, when necessary. Indeed, the first change she made was to break up with a boyfriend who had been holding her back for far too long. Also, she had some frank conversations with her mother, which led to Susan's gaining the personal distance from her that she had always needed. And when she finally let her father know she'd been running—a lot—he began to offer his daughter some running advice, which became the unlikely foundation for the relationship they had both wanted but had never been able to build before.

But the most striking of all the changes has been in Susan's enthusiasm for living. At the core of this transformation was a long-overdue reintegration of her body, mind, and spirit. "I began to own my body—to really love it and what it could do," she recalls of the period when she became a runner. She began to feel more beautiful and even to enjoy sex for the first time. Susan also began to enjoy food for the first time and to truly nourish her body with it. She took up cooking, which

Runner's Low

Endorphins are brain chemicals that produce feelings of well-being. They are released during prolonged and intense running and are believed to account for the so-called runner's high. But researchers have found that endorphin levels are abnormally low in runners suffering from overtraining syndrome, whose main symptom is an unexplained loss of performance but which is also characterized by depression. It is still unclear to what degree low endorphin levels are a cause or an effect of overtraining syndrome, but a general sense of lethargy and depression is frequently the very first symptom of the problem. Runners often look to performance or a miracle blood test to tell them when they are training too hard, when all they need to do is ask a close friend or a loved one whether they have seemed a little depressed, and they'll have their answer.

has become one of her favorite hobbies, and in fact she now hosts dinner parties regularly.

In general, now, Susan relishes life's familiar routines and chases after new experiences with a passion and joy that were sorely lacking in the past. As an athlete, she has expanded beyond running to hiking, climbing, yoga, and snowboarding. She has diversified her professional life to include work with a variety of people, from everyday folks who are unhappy to severe schizophrenics, and she is even writing a book. "Today," she says, "if you asked anyone who knows me to describe me in five words, they would all say 'adventurous.' Before I started running, nobody who knew me would have described me with that word. I'm proud of that. I'm enjoying being who I am."

The Great Mind Changer

Susan's inspiring story, although remarkable in its details, is very common in its general outline. In fact, you'd be hard pressed to find a runner whose mental health has not benefited noticeably in some way from running. How has running affected your mind? Has it reduced your stress level? Has it made you more focused and productive at work? Does it just put you in a better mood each day? Aerobic activities such as running are scientifically proven to provide such mental health benefits, among others.

When researchers began to discover these benefits in the 1960s, they were quite surprised. It seemed strange that activity of the body should have such powerful effects on the mind. Perhaps it still seems strange to you. The reason the mental health benefits of physical exercise are so counterintuitive for many is that we tend to forget that the mind is nothing more than the brain's way of experiencing itself, and the brain is as much a part of the body as the heart, the colon, and the kneecaps. This tendency to think of the mind (or the brain) and the body as separate is sometimes referred to as the "dualist fallacy." It is based on the false notion that thoughts, emotions, and such are not physical, when in fact they are physical.

Every sensation, thought, and emotion you experience is the result of a particular pattern of chemical and electrical activity in your brain. You can't have the experience without that pattern of activity, and whenever that pattern of activity does occur, you have that specific experience—even if the activity is artificially induced. For example, when brain researchers stimulate specific brain regions with small jolts of electricity, awake subjects often suddenly experience detailed memories, or smell strong odors, or burst out laughing or crying. These are the very brain regions that become active when a memory is spontaneously recalled, or a room with a strong odor is entered, or something funny or sad happens.

Chemical and electrical signals pass back and forth unceasingly between the brain and the rest of the body. That's why you can increase or decrease your running pace at will and feel your feet hitting the ground. It's also why running (and other forms of exercise) is able to change the brain, hence the mind, in the short term and the long term. For example, while you run, your body releases phenylalanine (PEA), a stimulatory neurotransmitter that increases mental activity and alertness. Because of this effect, people are generally able to concentrate better after exercise than at other times.

Many of the researchers who are discovering such effects believe there is a very simple evolutionary reason why running enhances brain health. The reason nervous systems exist in those creatures that have them is to enable movement. In primitive animals with rudimentary nervous systems that do not include a brain, movement control is the nervous system's only function. In the whole animal kingdom, humans have the most sophisticated nervous system, including the most complex brain, which is capable of doing much more than controlling movement. Yet everything our brains do is connected to movement, which remains job number one. More than one neuroscientist has called thought "the internalization of movement."

Half of the job of controlling movement is causing movement. The other half is receiving feedback from the body and environment during movement and adaptively recording this feedback to make future movement more effective. In other words, the nervous system learns movement through movement, so that the organism can more effectively find

The Mental Warmup

It's a scientifically proven fact that it's harder to solve challenging math problems while exercising intensely. That's because exercise robs fuel and oxygen from the parts of the brain that handle such tasks, ensuring that the motor centers are well supplied. But the brain is never sharper than it is after a run. After you run, your brain has elevated levels of chemicals, such as brain-derived neurotrophic factor, that enhance your ability to learn, remember, analyze, and compute. In a 2007 German study, people learned new words 20 percent faster after a workout than before a workout. So if you want to be as productive as possible at school or work, run first thing in the morning. It's the ultimate mental warmup.

food, flee danger, and so forth. Lower animals that cannot think in any fair sense of the word do all of their learning by moving. We humans aren't much different. Activity changes our brains. Physical exertion puts our brains in a state that is conducive to learning. Repeated physical exertion makes our brains generally better able to learn, function, and adapt by stimulating the growth of new cells, increasing the brain's fuel efficiency, and stimulating other changes that are very much like the exercise-induced changes we are familiar with in other organs, such the muscles. What's more, some of the very same changes that make our brains better able to learn also improve our moods, increase our capacity to handle stress, and enhance our self-esteem and all-around sense of well-being. Indeed, John Ratey, MD, one of the world's foremost experts on the effects of exercise on the brain, has written, "[Exercise] makes the brain function at its

best, and in my view, this effect of physical activity is far more important . . . than what it does for the body. Building muscles and conditioning the heart and lungs are essentially side effects."

Let's take a closer look at some of the specific brain health benefits of exercise.

Runner's High

When runners are surveyed about their motivations for running, enjoyment is invariably cited as the most important motivator. We become runners because we enjoy running. It feels good—not always, and never exclusively (it's almost always hard work), but enough to keep us coming back for more. So peculiar is this form of enjoyment to running that it even has its own name: the runner's high. What is it?

For some time the leading theoretical explanation of runner's high centered on endorphins: neurotransmitters that are produced during exercise and act on opioid receptors in the brain—the same receptors that various drugs, including morphine, act upon to produce feelings of well-being and euphoria. However, studies performed in the 1980s seemed to suggest that endorphins are at most only partly responsible for the joy of running; the runner's high was found to occur even when endorphin receptors were chemically blocked.

More recent research using advanced technologies has revitalized the endorphin theory. A team of researchers at Munich Technical University, led by Henning Boecker, used a technique called positron emission tomography (PET) scanning to measure endorphin levels and track the binding of endorphins to opioid receptors in areas of the brain associated with mood and emotion before and after a two-hour run. Ten runners were injected with chemical tracers to reveal the presence of endorphins through a PET scan. The runners underwent a baseline scan before the run and a follow-up scan immediately afterward.

Sure enough, after the run, the researchers found significantly increased levels of endorphins and reduced opioid receptor availability in specific brain regions associated with pleasure and emotions, including the limbic system and the prefrontal cortex. The 10 runners who participated in the study reported greatly increased feelings of euphoria after the run,

and those who felt most euphoric showed the highest levels of opioid receptor binding.

Beyond endorphins, exercise increases brain levels of entirely different classes of neurotransmitters that positively affect mood in other ways. Most important are norepinephrine, which increases alertness; dopamine, which elevates mood; and serotonin, the neurotransmitter that is most commonly targeted by antidepressants.

Neurotransmitters in general are unlikely to fully account for the joy of running. That's because, in addition to elevating the happy-making brain chemicals we've just mentioned, running also changes the rhythm of brain activity. Specifically, it induces a rhythmical pattern of neural firing known as the alpha-wave state, which is associated with feelings of calmness and well-being, also produced by meditation. Alpha rhythms, which are measured with electroencephalograph (EEG) sensors affixed to the head, indicate reduced activity in the higher processing centers of the brain. It has been proposed that increased activation of the brain's motor centers during exercise creates a competition for resources that deactivates the higher processing centers. This "empty-minded" state is experienced as peaceful and relaxed. Other types of research, including studies that track blood flow and metabolic patterns in the brain during exercise, have confirmed earlier EEG studies showing increased activity in the motor sensors and sharply reduced activity in the "thinking" parts of the brain.

It is important to point out that these biological changes associated with running enjoyment may be partly psychological in origin. Factors such as the feeling of accomplishment that comes with progressing through a workout and the pleasure of running in a beautiful natural environment on a sunny day are very likely to augment the purely physical brain changes that cause us to smile inwardly as we run.

Better than Prozac

If running's effects on mood were strictly acute—in other words, if they lasted only as long as the run itself did—they would still be quite valuable. But a consistent running habit actually produces a general increase in happiness. In fact, a growing number of psychiatrists believe that aerobic exercise is the best mood therapy available, as it has immediate effects and works for almost everyone, without negative side effects.

Consider a 2007 study performed by medical psychologist James Blumenthal, PhD, and his colleagues at Duke University Medical Center. One hundred and fifty-six men and women diagnosed with major depressive disorder were divided into three groups, which were treated with either exercise alone, medication (Zoloft) alone, or exercise and medication. After 16 weeks, 60.4 percent of the patients in the exercise group were no longer depressed, compared with 65.5 percent of those in the medication group and 68.8 percent of those in the combined group.

And that's not all. The more time passed, the better exercise fared against medication as a treatment for depression. After an additional six months, only 8 percent of the subjects who continued exercising became depressed again, while 38 percent of the medication group and 31 percent of the combined group relapsed. Blumenthal speculated that those in the exercise group might have fared better than those in the exercise-and-medication group because some members of the latter group were disappointed to learn that they were receiving medication instead of a placebo and consequently felt less "in control" of their progress than those who knew that exercise alone was responsible for their progress.

How does exercise treat depression so effectively? Scientists still don't know the whole story, but they have uncovered some parts of it. Most antidepressant medications work by increasing brain levels of neurotransmitters that have a positive effect on mood. Exercise, by wholly different mechanisms, increases the availability and effectiveness of the very same chemicals. Phil Holmes of the University of Georgia has shown that exercise

It Works Both Ways

Running makes you feel good, but feeling good also makes you run. This was shown in a study by Beth Lewis, PhD, an exercise and sports psychologist at the University of Minnesota. She had a group of sedentary adults complete a moderate-intensity workout and fill out a questionnaire designed to determine the workout's effect on their mood. The participants were then encouraged to maintain a regular exercise program. Lewis found that those who most enjoyed their first workout were significantly more likely to still be exercising 6 months later and 1 year later.

reduces depressive behaviors by increasing levels of norepinephrine, a neurotransmitter related to alertness and self-esteem, in certain parts of the brain. Interestingly, norepinephrine is also involved in learning through actions, and Holmes has shown that exercise regulates a gene that produces galanin, a neuropeptide that ensures that the right amount of norepinephrine is present at the right times to facilitate learning.

Exercise has also been shown to increase dopamine storage in the brain and to stimulate the development of new dopamine receptors in the brain's mood centers. And, not least of all, exercise boosts serotonin, the best-known mood-related neurotransmitter, which is also targeted by the best-known antidepressant medication, Prozac. Like norepinephrine, serotonin not only lifts mood and self-esteem but plays a role in learning as well. Specifically, it strengthens neural connections in the cerebral cortex and hippocampus, helping with memory formation.

Apart from its effects on neurotransmitters, exercise stimulates neurogenesis, the growth of new brain cells, which is another phenomenon that elevates mood and improves learning capacity. Depression is actually associated with atrophy in the prefrontal cortex and the hippocampus due to brain cell death. The popular antidepressant medications overcome this problem somewhat by increasing levels of neurotransmitters that facilitate the flow of information through the remaining neurons. But these drugs have limited capacity to grow new brain cells, whereas exercise exerts a powerful neurogenerative effect by increasing the production of compounds, including one called brain-derived neurotrophic factor, that play critical roles in the process.

Something for Everyone

You don't have to be clinically depressed to benefit from this effect of exercise. Exercise stimulates neurogenesis and boosts neurotransmitters in every person, not just those with diagnosable mood disorders. A 1993 study done in Athens found that mood remained slightly elevated in women 24 hours after a workout compared with controls who did not exercise. This finding suggests that if you run once a day, the mood-lifting benefit of your last run will just be wearing off when you begin your next one.

Furthermore, while only one in six people suffers from depression, everyone experiences stress, and running greatly increases the capacity of the brain and the rest of the body to manage stress. In so doing, running also greatly reduces the negative effects of stress on the brain and the rest of the body.

Stress is a complex physiological response to threats to the organism. A stressor is any type of threat, physical or psychological, that provokes this response. In modern life, most stressors are psychological in nature: near accidents on the freeway, deadline pressure at work, spousal disagreements, and so forth. But physical stressors are also common elements of modern life. These include inadequate sleep, hectic days without much opportunity to relax, and poor diet. Physical and psychological stressors affect the body in more or less the same way. Stress starts in the amygdala, the brain's most primitive fear center, which initiates the body's response to a perceived threat by sending out signals that increase heart rate, muscle tension, blood flow, and alertness. Other major coordinators of the stress response are the hypothalamus, which regulates basic body functions; the

Pull the Ripcord

Running doesn't reduce stress only in the long term. It's also an immediate stress reliever, as you probably already know. Scientists know it too. A number of studies have shown that a workout reduces the rise in blood pressure that is associated with psychosocial stressors. Such findings provide clear evidence of an instant mellowing effect of exercise. So whenever you're feeling a little too stressed out and want instant relief, go for a run. Some runners refer to this practice of running whenever and wherever necessary to relieve stress as "pulling the ripcord." Research indicates that either a slow half-hour run or a brisk shorter run will do the job.

pituitary gland; and the adrenal gland, which contributes to the stress response by releasing the hormones epinephrine (to prepare the muscles for action) and cortisol (to mobilize energy sources, among other things).

A little stress does no harm—in fact, a little stress is the very thing that strengthens the body's stress-management system, as Hans Selye showed and we discussed at the outset of this book. But chronic stress has major health consequences. When stress becomes chronic, cortisol levels are persistently elevated. Excess cortisol actually erodes brain connections, breaks down muscle tissue, and promotes visceral fat storage. Due to elevated cortisol and other biochemical imbalances, chronic stress increases the risk of anxiety, depression, diabetes, heart disease, Alzheimer's disease, and cancer.

Running is a stressor too, but unless you run too much, it is a positive stressor that limits the damage done by other stressors. It elevates your stress threshold, so your amygdala is not so easily triggered by perceived threats. Studies have shown, for example, that highly trained individuals release fewer inflammatory chemicals in response to mental stressors than unfit individuals. Running also reduces resting muscle tension, so that the body feels more relaxed. In addition, running increases the body's capacity to do everything it has to do when responding to stressors, from increasing blood flow to vital areas to releasing energy rapidly. Consequently, the stress response does not tax the fit body as much as it does the unfit body. Finally, running increases your body's ability to recover from stress by stimulating the growth of new brain cells to replace those killed off by stress and by causing your heart rate to return to normal faster, among other ways.

You're In Control

One of the important factors that make exercise different from other stressors is that you're in control of it. Not only does it make you feel good, but you know it makes you feel good, and you can do it whenever you want and also stop doing it whenever you want. This feeling of control is so very important. Research has shown that men and women who work in high-stress jobs in which they exercise a lot of control suffer fewer stress-related health consequences than men and women in equally high-stress jobs in which they lack control. Feeling in control of a stressful situation actually makes the situation less stressful. Knowing there's something you can do about the stress in your life increases what psychologists call your sense of self-efficacy, which is a major component of what the rest of us call happiness. Susan became a happier person when she took up running not only because of its biological effects on her brain, but also because it made her feel in control of how she felt for the first time since she was a small child.

PART 5

The Immune

System

Imagine for a moment that your body is a nation. Every nation has various governmental offices whose function is to protect it from external and internal threats. The armed forces ensure that enemy nations and terrorist organizations do not invade the country and wreak havoc. Customs and border protection works to distinguish those who belong within the nation's border and those who do not. The Federal Bureau of Investigation and other domestic law enforcement bodies protect the nation against threats originating within the nation's borders. In this analogy, your immune system is like the armed forces, customs and border protection, and FBI of your body.

The skin serves as your body's border patrol. It is a membrane that keeps the stuff that is you within and the stuff that is not you out. Beyond serving as a simple barrier, the skin contains various types of immune cells that detect viral and bacterial invaders and destroy them. But the skin is not the only possible point of entry of enemy invaders, or pathogens, into your body. Others include your respiratory tract and digestive tract. Your immune system has a sentry posted at every point where pathogens could gain access to your vital organs. Your respiratory tract secretes germ-killing peptides, while your digestive organs contain germ-killing enzymes and also host friendly bacteria that combat unfriendly bacteria.

To the degree that these surface barriers fail, your body relies on the innate immune system to identify and destroy the invaders. The major workhorses of the innate immune system are the white blood cells, of which there are many types. The "first responders" are a type called macrophages, which dismantle or engulf pathogens and then send chemical signals that call other types to the scene.

A number of internal organs have immune functions. The thymus is a gland in the upper chest that incubates T cells and other immune cells. The bone marrow is another site of immune cell production. The spleen, a small organ in the abdomen, processes pathogens and produces specific antibodies to them. An antibody (or immunoglobulin) is like a special protein key that fits the lock of individual pathogens. The lymphatic system is a network of fluid-containing nodes that collect the waste material from infections and drain it from the body.

A properly functioning immune system is critical to life and health. It is also critical to running performance. Running challenges the immune system in a number of ways. To begin with, a single hard run temporarily suppresses immune function, increasing the body's susceptibility to infection. The causes

of this effect appear to be multiple and are not fully understood; but part of the problem is that the immune cells' main fuels, such as the amino acid glutamine, are depleted during strenuous exercise. It seems the immune system also downgrades its inflammatory response to tissue damage to avoid out-of-control systemic inflammation that would otherwise result from the high muscle damage caused by exercise. But this very reduction in response impairs the immune system's ability to fight foreign invaders.

Overall, however, running strengthens the immune system. Moderate exercise stimulates a temporary increase in the production of macrophages. The more fit a person becomes, the longer these transient bumps last, until the positive effect is essentially continuous in the daily exerciser. The benefits go far beyond fewer colds and flus. Many cases of autoimmune disease, such as rheumatoid arthritis, are triggered by infections, so running may reduce the risk of such conditions. Infections are also fingered as initial culprits in the development of chronic diseases such as atherosclerosis, whose risk is known to be sharply reduced by aerobic exercise. A strong immune system also helps fight cancer, and there is increasing evidence that aerobic fitness provides protection against a variety of cancer types.

Heavy exercise is itself a physiological stressor that provokes a protective (and adaptive) immune response. Without a properly functioning immune system, you could not recover from your daily runs. A smart approach to training will enhance the immune system activities that allow you to recover and adapt to training, but an over-zealous approach will overwhelm your immune system, resulting in injuries and declining performance. We recommend the smart approach!

Chapter 14

Radicals and Inflamers

The late 19th-century German philosopher Friedrich Nietzsche famously wrote, "That which does not kill me makes me stronger." The profound general truth of this statement has been recognized since Nietzsche's contemporaries first read it. But thanks to a recent turn in the field of biology, it seems truer now than ever.

The biological parallel of Nietzsche's statement is the principle of *hormesis*. This principle has been around for decades, but only recently has it begun to gain widespread acceptance. The basic premise of hormesis is that bodily influences that are toxic in large doses are often beneficial in small doses. More specifically, in small doses, many, if not most, toxic influences stress the body just enough to provoke an adaptive response that boosts the body's ability to manage future exposures to the same type of stressor.

Examples of hormesis are everywhere. Nutritional examples include vitamins A and B_6, selenium, iron, and zinc, all of which are essential for life but are toxic at high doses. The benefits of exercise are also partially hormetic in nature. For example, the muscle fuel depletion that occurs during exercise stimulates a stress response pathway that increases the muscles' ability to take up glucose in response to insulin. This adaptation increases the body's capacity to store fuel for future exercise, which boosts exercise ability and reduces the risk of diabetes.

Hormesis is also fundamental to the workings of the human immune system. When a virus invades your body, your immune system responds by creating antibodies specifically designed to eliminate that particular virus. As a result, after you get rid of it, the virus can never again make you sick. This is why most vaccines consist of small doses of the very viruses that they are supposed to inoculate you against. That which doesn't kill you makes you stronger.

The principle of hormesis in relation to exercise and the immune system affects the way the body handles damage to the muscles and other tissues that occurs during running. The job of limiting and reversing this wear and tear falls to your body's inflammatory response and antioxidant defense system. The inflammatory response initiates tissue repair after damage has already been done. The antioxidant defense system consists of a complex network of compounds that help to prevent tissue damage caused by free radicals, or unstable molecules produced as products of muscle metabolism. As we will see in this chapter, through hormesis, running strengthens both your inflammatory response and your antioxidant defense system, making you less susceptible to running-induced tissue damage and better able to recover from it. As a result, your running performance increases, and you can handle a greater training load.

Hormesis is always a double-edged sword, however. It works in your favor only when the dosage of a particular toxic influence is large enough to have an effect but not so large that it overwhelms your defenses. Inflammation has a way of becoming out of control in runners who train too much and rest too little, causing a downward spiral in performance. In other words, when the "dosage" of running is too high, inflammation changes from a positive to a negative.

Similarly, although free radicals cause muscle damage during running, they are also the primary stimulus for strengthening the antioxidant defense system. There is evidence that thwarting free radical production too much—for example, by consuming large quantities of antioxidant supplements—might attenuate some of the normal benefits of training. In other words, when the dosage of free radicals is artificially limited, antioxidants change from a good thing to a bad thing.

What's more, the inflammatory response itself produces free radicals that aid in the cleanup process at the site of tissue damage. Running actually increases the free radical production capacity of certain types of white blood cells that participate in the inflammatory response, and that's a good thing. But again, when inflammation gets out of hand, so does free radical production, and as a result, the very process that is supposed to help repair tissue damage causes more damage.

Are you confused? Perhaps, and that is okay, as we are dealing with concepts that are both abstract and physiologically complex. Don't worry, though, because the bottom line is quite simple: Muscle damage, free radicals, antioxidant defenses, and inflammation can all help or hurt your running. Let's see what you can do to ensure that they don't kill you but make you stronger!

Free Radicals, Antioxidants, and Muscle Damage

Oxygen is considered a reactive element because it contains two unpaired electrons, and electrons like to pair with other electrons. Therefore oxygen is prone to form bonds with other molecules that also have electrons to share. It's no accident that oxygen is the atmospheric element that our bodies absorb for use in the metabolic reactions that power us.

Our muscles use more oxygen than any other organ in our body, especially when we're running. Within muscle cells, oxygen receives electrons from carbohydrate, fat, and, to a lesser degree, amino acid molecules through a complex process that we described generally in Part 3. This process produces molecules of ATP, which is the only direct source of energy for muscle contractions. A small fraction of the electrons that are transferred in this multistep process leak out and form free radicals, such as nitric oxide and superoxide, which quickly turns into hydrogen peroxide. These two major muscle-generated free radicals are able to pass outside cell membranes, but many other minor types cannot, so we know much less about them. Inherently unstable, these free radicals "steal" electrons from other molecules, increasing their own stability at the cost of damage to cellular components and the cre-ation of new free radicals, resulting in a chain reaction.

Because the rate of oxygen consumption increases dramatically during exercise, the rate of oxygen free radical production in the working muscles also increases. However, recent research suggests that the increase is not nearly as great as was once believed and that a majority of the free radicals produced by the muscles during exercise are generated by other mechanisms. Scientists used to think of free radical production during exercise as a sort of accidental by-product of metabolism with strictly negative conse-quences (the main consequence being muscle tissue damage). Now it is seen as an integral component of muscle metabolism that is closely regulated. We have learned that some free radicals trigger changes in muscle cell signaling that in turn stimulate some of the muscles' positive fitness adaptations to exercise—hormesis at work. In particular, free radical production during exercise acti-vates the genes that govern the antioxidant defenses, rendering the muscles better able to limit free radical production in future runs.

The primary form of free radical damage that muscle cells suffer during running is lipid peroxidation, which occurs when elec-trons are pilfered from the fats in cell mem-branes. Disruption of a cell's membrane causes some of its contents, including enzymes such as creatine kinase (CK), to leak into the extracellular space. Exercise scientists measure creatine kinase levels in the blood after exercise to gauge the amount of muscle damage caused by the workout. In a recovered state, the typical runner's serum creatine kinase level is approximately 125 units per liter (U/L). Twenty-four hours after completion of a half-marathon, the CK level doubles. One day after a full marathon, CK levels in recreational runners are roughly 15 times normal. (The change is less dramatic in highly trained competitive runners.) And the average CK level in a runner who has just completed the 135-mile Badwater Ultramarathon is 3,570 U/L, more than 28 times the resting value. That's a lot of leaky muscle cells.

Defending the Castle

The antioxidant defenses within muscle cells prevent muscle damage resulting from free radical production from becoming even worse. These defenses consist of enzymes such as superoxide dismutase and glutathione peroxidase, as well as the antioxidants glutathione, vitamin E, and vitamin C. Slow-twitch muscle fibers—the endurance specialists—contain greater concentrations of antioxidants, because they also produce the most free radicals. As mentioned above, in a shining example of hormesis, exercise training bolsters the muscles' antioxidant defenses by challenging them with free radical production. Many of the free radicals generated during exercise act as signals that communicate with DNA through intermediaries such as protein kinase, activated by mitogen (a chemical substance, usually some form of a protein, that promotes the commencement of cell division). These intermediaries enhance the expression of genes that govern antioxidant defense activity.

Numerous studies have shown that exercise increases the antioxidant capacity of the muscles. For example, in one study, a group of untrained individuals performed cycling tests to exhaustion before and after completing a challenging 12-week running program. The researchers found that lipid peroxidation resulting from the cycling test was significantly lower after the training period.

Free Radicals, Antioxidants, and Fatigue

Many runners already know that free radicals produced during running cause muscle damage. But most are not aware that free radicals may also contribute to fatigue. Again, there is a beneficial hormetic effect to be had. Just as free radicals not only cause muscle damage but also help prevent it by stimulating a strengthening of the muscles' antioxidant defenses, free radicals also help the muscles become more fatigue-resistant through the same stimulating influence.

During short, moderate-intensity exercise, free radicals produced by working muscles actually assist muscle work by facilitating glucose transport into muscle cells. But when free radicals are produced at high levels during prolonged or intense exercise, they begin to inhibit muscle work. Free radicals appear to cause fatigue, at least in part, by reducing calcium sensitivity in muscle cell proteins. Calcium ions play a key role in transmitting motor nerve impulses within muscle cells. When the muscle cell proteins become less calcium sensitive, muscle fiber is no longer able to contract as forcefully, and performance declines.

The primary antioxidant in muscle cells is glutathione, which neutralizes free radicals and thereby mitigates their negative effects on muscle work. Through this process, however, glutathione eventually becomes depleted, at which point the muscles' antioxidant system is unable to delay fatigue any longer. This raises an obvious question: Can antioxidant-rich foods or supplements enhance glutathione stores and thereby increase endurance? Scientists have studied the effects of infusion and ingestion of various compounds that regenerate glutathione in hopes that they might further delay free radical–induced muscle fatigue. At the same time, scientists are also actively studying the possible performance-enhancing effects of antioxidants that may work by other mechanisms.

To date there has been no research on the effects of antioxidant-rich foods (i.e., fruits and vegetables) on exercise fatigue. We do know, however, that a diet rich in fruits and vegetables increases the body's overall antioxidant capacity—and the muscle cells' ability to limit the fatigue-inducing effects of free radical production during exercise is a big part of that overall capacity. So you have yet another potential reason to eat your fruits and vegetables!

A scoring system known as the oxygen radical absorbance capacity (ORAC) is used to rate the antioxidant capacity of foods. The accompanying table lists the ORAC scores of a number of antioxidant-rich fruits and vegetables. These foods should be mainstays in your diet.

Interestingly, new research suggests that it might not be the antioxidants per se in fruits and vegetables that increase the antioxidant capacity of people who consume them. Indeed, most antioxidants in the concentrations normally found in fruits and vegetables are not potent enough to scavenge meaningful amounts of free radicals. Antioxidants are part of a wider class of plant nutrients called phytochemicals, many of which are toxic at high doses. But at the low doses found in fruits and vegetables, these toxins provoke a mild stress response in the cell that increases its own built-in antioxidant defenses. In other words, certain foods may enhance the body's antioxidant capacity—and the muscle

Fruits	ORAC Value	Vegetables	ORAC Value
Prunes	5,770	Kale	1,770
Raisins	2,830	Spinach, raw	1,260
Blueberries	2,400	Brussels sprouts	980
Blackberries	2,036	Alfalfa sprouts	930
Cranberries	1,750	Spinach, steamed	909
Strawberries	1,540	Broccoli florets	890
Pomegranates	1,245	Beets	841
Raspberries	1,220	Red bell pepper	713
Plums	949	Onion	450
Oranges	750	Corn	400
Grapes, red	739	Eggplant	390
Cherries	670	Cauliflower	377
Kiwifruit	602	Peas, frozen	364
Grapes, white	446	White potatoes	313
Cantaloupe	252	Sweet potatoes	301
Banana	221	Carrots	207
Apple	218	String beans	201
Apricots	164	Tomato	189
Peach	158	Zucchini	176
Pear	134	Yellow squash	150

Source: Agriculture Research, 1999

damage reduction and fatigue resistance that come with it—in the same way exercise does: through hormesis.

What happens if we extract one or more of the nontoxic or less-toxic antioxidant phytonutrients from plants and consume them supplementally? Many antioxidant supplements are potent enough to measurably supplement the body's built-in antioxidant defenses. And some may even delay fatigue and enhance endurance performance. For example, there is cause to believe that a class of antioxidants called phytoestrogens has performance-boosting potential when consumed supplementally. Phytoestrogens are found in greatest abundance in nuts, seeds, and soy products. In a recent scientific paper, researchers at the University of Valencia, Spain, proposed that phytoestrogens might enhance the expression of the genes that govern the body's antioxidant defenses, just as exercise itself does.

The difference between antioxidants that directly neutralize free radicals in the body and those such as phytoestrogens, that build up the body's innate capacity to produce anti-oxidants could be an important one. As we've mentioned, one major benefit of free radical production by the working muscles during exercise is that it stimulates physiological

The Trouble with Pills

When you think of treatments for inflammation, the first that come to mind are probably nonsteroidal anti-inflammatory drugs (NSAIDs). such as ibuprofen and aspirin. These over-the-counter medications are adequate for temporary relief from the symptoms of severe pain and inflammation due to injury. However, they are not a good choice to treat the delayed-onset muscle soreness (DOMS) and inflammation that you experience as normal conse-quences of hard training. There are five major problems with NSAIDs:

1. *Ulcers.* By reducing production of key prostaglandins (hormonelike compounds manufac-tured in the body) that protect the stomach lining, long-term use of some NSAIDs can cause ulcers to develop.

2. *Kidney damage.* Over the long-term, some NSAIDs also reduce production of prostaglan-dins that promote blood flow to the kidneys, which may eventually lead to kidney damage.

3. *Joint cartilage damage.* Long-term use of a few NSAIDs (including ibuprofen) has been shown to cause joint cartilage degeneration.

4. *Slower muscle protein synthesis after exercise.* Research has shown that ibuprofen and acetaminophen (Tylenol) slow the process of muscle protein synthesis after exercise. Postexercise muscle protein synthesis is critical to muscle regeneration after workouts.

5. *Impaired healing processes.* As discussed in Chapter 2, the inflammatory process is actually a crucial component of the recovery process. Similarly, after acute injuries, inflammation is vital because it helps to clear away damaged tissue, effectively creating space for the rebuilding of healthy tissue where the damage occurred. Interfering with this process is likely to compromise the long-term prognosis, and so the early stages of inflammation are important on the journey to recovery. Only if the inflammation becomes prolonged and excessive should steps be taken to reduce it.

adaptations that strengthen the body's anti-oxidant defenses. In other words, the free radical damage that occurs during exercise has a training effect that results in stronger antioxidant defenses, much as glycogen depletion during exercise stimulates a greater capacity for glycogen storage and fat-burning. The Spanish research team mentioned above has pointed out that antioxidants that interfere with free radical production during exercise inhibit these beneficial adaptations. That is, they act as a sort of crutch. So it's possible that certain antioxidant supplements might do more harm than good. But phytoestrogens are one example of a type of antioxidant that seems to act as a kick in the pants, rather than a crutch, to the muscles' built-in antioxidant defenses.

Again, we will have to wait for science to take a few steps forward before we can sort out which specific types of antioxidant supplementation (if any) are truly beneficial and which are counterproductive.

How Inflammation Works

As we suggested at the beginning of the chapter, the body's antioxidant defenses and its inflammatory response are interrelated. That's because the free radicals that slip through the muscles' antioxidant defenses to cause cell damage trigger the inflammatory response, whose job is to initiate the process of repairing the damage. Antioxidant defenses

are like a building's sprinkler system that turns on to protect the building at the first sign of smoke. The inflammatory response is like the fire department that comes to douse the blaze after it has overwhelmed the sprinkler system.

We met the inflammatory process as the culprit responsible for the symptoms you experience after your first run, or after an unaccustomed hard bout of training that causes DOMS (Chapter 2). You are probably accustomed to thinking of inflammation as an obvious swelling, stiffening, and warming of the tissues around an injured joint, but a milder inflammatory response occurs after every run. Any part of your anatomy that is sore the day after a run is likely to host some inflammatory activity. Most of the tissue damage that receives attention from the inflammatory response after a run is caused not by free radicals, however, but instead by simple mechanical stress. For example, a muscle fiber tries to shorten at the same time gravity tries to stretch it, and it ruptures.

The inflammatory response has three overlapping phases. First, blood accumulates at the site of damage. This causes the classic symptoms of swelling, heat, and stiffness associated with inflammation. Next, specialized white blood cells called neutrophils migrate to the injured area and absorb the debris of damaged cells. Finally, other cells known as macrophages accumulate at the site of damage to complete the cleanup process

Isn't That Swell?

The type of swelling that occurs in a sore knee after a run is known as acute, or local, inflammation. There's also another, very different type of inflammation, known as chronic, or systemic, inflammation. Systemic inflammation is inflammation of the blood and/or artery walls caused by bacterial infection and other factors, such as free radicals and high levels of blood lipids. Systemic inflammation is closely linked to atherosclerosis, or the stiffening of arteries through the formation of fatty plaques. When free radical–damaged blood lipids or other factors create a lesion in the artery walls, an inflammatory response results. As such lesions accumulate, inflammation becomes chronic and actually accelerates the formation of fatty plaques that stiffen the arteries, increasing the risk of heart attack and stroke.

Inflammation is also linked to diabetes. A study by researchers at Brigham and Women's Hospital in Boston found that those with the highest blood levels of two inflammatory compounds—interleukin-6 and C-reactive protein—were six times more likely to develop type 2 diabetes than women with low levels of the compounds. Even Alzheimer's disease and some cancers have an apparent inflammation link.

The good news is that exercise significantly reduces systemic inflammation. Most notably, exercise reduces the blood concentration of C-reactive protein. It appears that the repeated low-grade inflammatory response that exercisers experience after workouts stimulates a larger increase in the production of anti-inflammatory compounds and antioxidant defenses, which protect against systemic inflammation (another case of hormesis, or the principle of "that which doesn't kill me makes me stronger," at work). One study by researchers at Auburn University found that markers of systemic inflammation were 76 percent lower in subjects with a high aerobic fitness level than in moderately fit counterparts. This is one reason why runners are much less likely than nonrunners to suffer heart attacks and strokes.

and stimulate tissue regeneration. (This process, relative to DOMS, was described in detail in Chapter 2.)

The locations and degrees of inflammation that follow a run depend on the speed and duration of the run, the fitness level of the runner, and the runner's anatomical structure and biomechanics. If a run is faster and/or longer than average, it will cause more tissue damage and therefore more inflammation. The fitter you are, the faster and longer you will have to run before you experience a significant degree of inflammation. Training increases the resistance of the muscles and joint tissues to the damage that precipitates inflammation.

Finally, inflammation will concentrate in areas of your body that are most susceptible to tissue damage during running. In all runners, the muscles and connective tissues that experience the most eccentric strain—where the muscle or connective tissue tries to shorten as the force of gravity attempts to lengthen it—will undergo the most disruption and subsequent inflammation. The quadriceps (especially in runs with substantial downhill portions) and Achilles tendons are on this list. Individual structural and biomechanical factors may cause tissue damage and inflammation to concentrate more in particular areas of one runner's body than another's. For example, female runners with broad hips are more likely to develop patellofemoral pain syndrome, which is now believed to be primarily an inflammatory condition.

It is not possible, nor would it be beneficial, to completely prevent postrun tissue inflammation. To begin with, the mild inflammation that follows a typical workout triggers adaptations that enhance your body's ability to limit and control inflammation in future runs. What's more, every runner, no matter how gifted and fit, must perform workouts that are faster and/or longer than normal to become fitter, and inflammation is an unavoidable effect of such workouts. The only

things you really need to do to limit postrun inflammation are the things you do to prevent injuries and overtraining generally: namely, increase your training load slowly and gradually, intersperse harder workouts with easier workouts in your training regimen, and take days off or cross-train when you experience unusual soreness in one or more areas.

Maintaining a healthy diet will also help your body manage inflammation better. Some nutrients, when consumed in excess, tend to increase production of pro-inflammatory cytokines and other compounds, while others limit their production. Studies have shown that diets high in starches, sugars, saturated fat, and trans fat are associated with high levels of systemic inflammation markers. Diets high in natural antioxidants and fiber, including moderate amounts of alcohol and caffeine and a balanced ratio of omega-6 and omega-3 fats, are associated with low levels of inflammation.

Specific foods believed to increase inflammation include processed meats and sugar-sweetened beverages. Foods that may reduce inflammation include fruits and vegetables, whole grain foods, soy foods, and good sources of omega-3 fats, such as salmon and flaxseeds.

The so-called Mediterranean diet happens to be heavy on anti-inflammatory foods (and beverages) and light on pro-inflammatory foods. The important components of this diet are fruits and vegetables, seafood, olive oil, and red wine. A study by researchers at the University of Athens, Greece, looked at the relationship between the Mediterranean diet and levels of C-reactive protein and other inflammatory biomarkers. This research was done as part of the ATTICA study, which tracked the eating patterns of more than 3,000 men and women over a two-year period. The study found that participants who stuck most closely to the traditional Mediterranean diet had, on average, 20 percent lower C-reactive protein levels, 14 percent lower white blood cell counts, 17 percent lower interleukin-6 levels, 6 percent lower fibrinogen levels, and 15 percent lower homocysteine levels compared with those who adhered the least to the Mediterranean diet.

Fish consumption alone accounted for many of these differences. Inflammation markers were as much as one-third lower in those individuals who ate at least 10 ounces of fish each week. Naturally, fish that are rich in omega-3 fats, such as wild salmon, herring, and mackerel, are especially beneficial.

Perhaps the most effective dietary measure you can adopt to reduce systemic inflammation is to avoid overeating and thus maintain a lean body composition. That's because fat cells produce inflammatory cytokines that stimulate the production of C-reactive protein. Different levels of body fat, especially in the abdomen, account for a sizable fraction of individual differences in systemic inflammation. So anything you can do dietwise to reduce your body fat percentage will also reduce your inflammation level.

Inflammation, Free Radicals, and Overtraining

In 2000, Lucille Lakier Smith, a sports scientist at Tshwane University of Technology in South Africa, proposed an explanation for overtraining syndrome that became known as the cytokine hypothesis. According to this hypothesis, overtraining syndrome—a condition affecting athletes in heavy training that is characterized by an unexpected deterioration of performance and a long list of hormonal, immunological, neurological, and psychological signs and symptoms—is triggered by the repetitive trauma that the muscles and connective tissues undergo during training. If severe training stress is imposed too frequently for the tissues to heal, chronic systemic inflammation will result. Cytokines are immune system messenger cells that coordinate this response, interacting with the endocrine and nervous systems to produce the other classic symptoms of overtraining syndrome, which include depression, sleep disturbance, poor immune function, and high levels of stress hormones.

Remember Selye's General Adaptation Principle? In her paper on the cytokine hypothesis of overtraining, Lakier Smith wrote, "Theoretically, [overtraining syndrome] is viewed as the third stage of Selye's General Adaptation Principle, with the focus being on recovery/survival, and not adaptation, and is deemed to be 'protective,' occurring in response to excessive physical/physiological stress." In this view, overtraining is the body's way of refusing to continue training at the level that is causing it to break down.

In reality, it's unlikely that something as complex as overtraining syndrome can be explained by one single hypothesis. Science has searched for the "magic bullet" to overtraining for perhaps 40 years and has not yet discovered it. Lakier Smith's cytokine hypothesis certainly seems to represent part, but not all, of the picture, and the theory has been validated by some research. For example, if systemic inflammation does underlie overtraining syndrome, we would expect to see high levels of oxidative stress and compromised antioxidant defenses in overtrained athletes, because inflammation generates a lot of free radicals. And in fact that is exactly what we do see, but it is impossible to tell whether that is a cause or an effect of the syndrome. Also, a variety of other biochemical abnormalities are also seen in overtrained athletes, as well as neurological, hormonal, and psychological changes, which emphasizes that while chronic inflammation might be one cause of overtraining syndrome,

current thinking leans toward the view that there is no single root cause of overtraining syndrome. Excessive exercise may stress any of a variety of physiological systems to the point of maladaptation, and as soon as one system reaches this point, a cascade effect that throws other systems out of balance is sure to follow.

So how do you know if you're among the ranks of the overtrained? The primary sign to look for is an unexpected decline in workout performance. Other symptoms include persistent fatigue, muscle soreness, and a loss of motivation for training. Often, the first symptoms are psychological—moodiness, depression, irritability, and frustration. Recent novel work has focused on developing mood assessment questionnaires and understanding how the mental and emotional states may predict the development of subsequent physiological overtraining. Another very common symptom is insomnia, which is often a very early symptom. Training should help athletes sleep more, but at some point it seems to produce the opposite effect, possibly by way of effects on the nervous system.

The cure for overtraining is relative rest—that is, reducing your training load until you begin to feel and perform better. But here are four training tactics that can help head off the downward spiral of overtraining.

Train progressively. The surest way to avoid overtraining is not to train very hard. But that's also the surest way not to get very fit. To build peak fitness without overtraining, you need to train progressively, or increase your training load at a gradual rate that stays within your body's adaptive limits. As a general rule, you should increase your weekly training volume by no more than 10 percent each week. So if you train 10 hours this week, train no more than 11 hours next week.

It is also important that you be conservative when increasing the amount of high-intensity training (lactate-threshold intensity and above) that you do each week. This is perhaps the most dangerous period of training: the point at which higher-intensity training is introduced. For example, the greatest amount of work at lactate threshold intensity you'd want to do in a single session is about 40 minutes. But if you haven't done threshold-intensity training recently, your first such workout should feature only 15 minutes or so at that intensity level. Try 18 minutes in your next threshold workout, and then 20, and so on.

Employ the hard-easy rule. The next workout you do after any challenging workout should be relatively easy, so that it won't interfere with your recovery. As a runner, designate three workouts per week (two high-intensity sessions and one long endurance session) as hard workouts. The rest should be easy to moderate. Here's a sample schedule:

Mon	Tue	Wed	Thu	Fri	Sat	Sun
Rest	Hard (high-intensity)	Easy	Easy	Hard (high-intensity)	Easy	Hard (long endurance)

Plan recovery weeks. Although your training should be progressive, it should not be progressive in the sense that it steadily and *continually* increases in volume. Instead, periodically intersperse brief periods of reduced training into your training progression to give your body a chance to fully absorb and recover from recent hard workouts and prepare for even harder workouts in the following weeks. We recommend that you plan every third or fourth week as a recovery week. Reduce your training volume by roughly 20 percent in these weeks, and do not include any hard running.

Listen to your body. If your training schedule is challenging enough to push you toward a true fitness peak, there will inevitably be times when you feel unexpectedly run-down. When this happens, heed the warning your body is giving you and take a day off, or at least replace your next hard workout with an easier one. Many competitive athletes find it difficult to pull back and allow for recovery in response to unexpected moments of accumulating fatigue, but it is usually the best choice. If you practice restraint and take it easy today, you will probably feel strong again tomorrow or the next day. But if you stubbornly persist in training hard despite your body's warnings, you may dig yourself deep into the hole of overtraining and find that it takes many weeks or even months to climb back out.

Chapter 15

Outrunning Illness

The average person comes down with two or three colds and flu infections each year. As a runner, you're far from average, and you're likely to have fewer infections than your couch-bound counterparts, as we shall see. But even one poorly timed cold or flu can wreak havoc on a runner's efforts to develop race fitness. Indeed, most bouts of illness are poorly timed for runners, because the stress of heavy training weakens the immune defenses and increases the odds of getting sick. Consequently, runners all too often find that they are able to train least effectively when they are trying to train the most seriously.

A typical case study involves two-time Olympian Dathan Ritzenhein. While preparing to defend his 2005 U.S. National Cross-Country Championship title, Ritzenhein began logging heavy miles at the height of cold and flu season (as the elite cross-country season arrives in the winter). A few weeks before the race, he caught what he thought was a garden variety chest cold. Since he had successfully "trained through" such illnesses in the past, he tried to do the same this time; not only did his symptoms linger, however, but his workout performances worsened. When race day arrived, he felt sluggish from the gun and finished a disappointing fourth.

After the race, Ritzenhein was diagnosed with walking pneumonia and ordered to cut back his training until he had fully recovered. The following year, 2007, he took greater precautions to protect his health and reclaimed the national championship in cross-country.

Let this story be a lesson to you! Good health is the foundation of productive training and successful racing. Running helps you stay in good health by strengthening the immune system so that it's better able to ward off viral invaders. But it will never ward off all of them, and when you do get sick, the best way to continue to put your running first is to put your health first. That's because hard running weakens an immune system that is already taxed by a battle against a viral infection, thereby prolonging the illness and sabotaging your running. What's more, even when you're healthy, especially hard workouts and races suppress the immune system and increase the risk of contracting infections, so it's important that during times when you need to train hard, you take every other precaution to stay healthy.

Exercise and the Immune System

Doctors and other healers have recognized the beneficial effects of physical exercise on the risk of illness for many centuries, but not until the past 150 years has it been understood that the immune system mediated these effects. In 1711, the English essayist and poet Joseph Addison wrote, "Exercise ferments the humors, casts them into their proper channels, throws off redundancies, and helps nature in those secret distributions, without which the body cannot subsist in its vigor, nor the soul act with cheerfulness." Not quite, Mr. Addison!

Today we know that exercise enhances the body's ability to "subsist in vigor" not by "fer-menting the humors" but instead by—well, to tell the truth, there's still a lot we don't know about how exercise enhances the body's resistance to viral infection. The major components of the innate system that is charged with identifying and destroying viruses include macrophages (which dismantle viral cells), cytokines (which are key signaling molecules of the immune system), and natural killer cells (whose name describes their function rather well). Research has shown that exercise changes these immune system components and others in ways that enable them to perform their functions more effectively.

Let's consider the specific example of heat shock proteins. Heat shock proteins are molecules released by the body in response to all types of stress, from exposure to high temperatures to viral infections to exercise. The increased production of heat shock proteins that occurs during exercise stimulates some of the body's fitness-boosting adaptive responses to training, because certain heat shock proteins are known to participate in muscle tissue remodeling. Some heat shock proteins are also known to bind to antigens, or foreign invaders, and chaperone them to the immune system. It now appears that the boost in heat shock protein activity that is caused by training not only increases fitness but also enhances the capacity of the heat shock proteins to respond to other stressors, including viral infections.

That's one simplified example. The effects of exercise on the immune system extend far beyond the heat shock proteins and indeed far beyond the limits of current scientific knowledge. What we do know with certainty is that moderate exercise reduces the frequency and severity of viral infections. One of the world's leading researchers on exercise and the immune system is David Nieman of Appalachian State University. In a 1993 study, Nieman put 16 previously sedentary women on a 23-week walking program and allowed 16 others to continue loafing around for comparison. During the study period, 21 percent of the walkers developed upper respiratory tract infections (URTIs), while 50 percent of the non-exercisers did. What's more, the rate of URTI in an age-matched group of highly trained runners over the same period of time was just 8 percent.

As we stated previously, however, athletes who maintain very heavy training workloads are as likely as loafers, or even more likely than loafers, to get sick. The reason is that

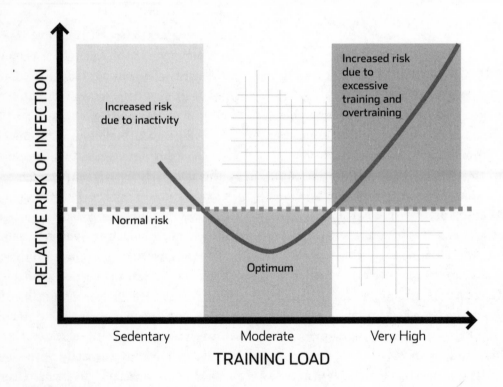

The relationship between the risk of illness and training load

exercise itself is a stressor that challenges the immune system. During periods of heavy training, the immune system is stretched to the limit trying to help the body recover between workouts, and there is no capacity left to fight illnesses. The risk is highest for runners who are overtraining to the point of performance decline during the period immediately after a longer race. For example, Nieman found that nearly 13 percent of participants in the 1990 Los Angeles Marathon got sick during the following week, compared with just 2.2 percent of runners who entered the race but did not participate for reasons other than illness.

The relationship between the risk of illness and training load is shown in the figure opposite. There is an "optimal" amount of exercise (with respect to both intensity and volume) at which risk is reduced; on either side of this optimum, the risk increases. Both loafers and overtrainers are more likely to get sick. Of course, defining "optimal" is the challenge—what is moderate for one person may be completely excessive for another, so one must use discretion to determine where that cutoff point might be.

Preventing Cold and Flu

One of the most effective things a runner in heavy training for an event can do to reduce the risk of getting sick is to reduce his or her training. This tactic is not acceptable to most competitive runners, however, because the reason they are training hard to begin with is to perform as well as possible in a race. While training less may prevent them from getting sick, it is almost certain to reduce their running performance level, unless they were overtraining to begin with. It is important to note that the increased susceptibility to cold and flu that comes with heavy training is not necessarily a sign of overtraining. In most cases, training has a mildly suppressive effect on the immune system at a level far below that at which true symptoms of overtraining, such as performance decline and severely compromised immune function, occur.

Many runners wrongly believe that they can reduce their risk of catching a cold or flu by bundling up before they run outdoors on cold or wet days or by not running at all in such weather. Despite tireless myth-busting efforts made by the medical community, the myth that exposure to cold and damp weather causes illnesses persists. But cold and flu viruses are always acquired, either directly or indirectly, through other affected people. So while you should always dress for maximum comfort when running outdoors in the winter, your chances of catching a cold while running alone in a blizzard are next to zero. It's much more likely that you will pick up a bug while sitting comfortably in a crowded room warmed by a roaring central heating system.

Because cold and flu viruses are always acquired through affected people, the surest way to avoid getting sick is to avoid other people, effectively placing yourself in quarantine! If you have a large and close extended family or work as a second-grade teacher, there is only so much you can do to avoid other people and their germs. However, there may be some specific measures you can take to limit your exposure. For example, you can politely put off social interaction with friends and relatives who are currently sick. Watch movies at home instead of in the theater during periods of heavy training that coincide with cold and flu season, and avoid taking unnecessary airplane flights. When you're trying to train hard through the winter, perhaps you can even telecommute to work some days.

It's possible to reduce the risk of being infected even when in the presence of those who already are. Infection is as likely to occur through direct physical contact with germs as it is through breathing contaminated air. Frequently washing your hands with soap and water (especially after touching "public" items such as doorknobs), avoiding handshakes, and keeping your hands away from your face will reduce the likelihood of your becoming infected in this manner.

While there may never be a cure for the common cold, there are vaccines for most strains of the flu virus, and if you are serious about minimizing sickness-induced interruptions to your training, you should get a flu shot or nasal spray inoculation before each flu season. They are 70 to 90 percent effective, and they cost little in terms of time, effort, or money. Call your physician to schedule a flu vaccination between September and November in the Northern Hemisphere and March and April in the Southern Hemisphere.

Running When You're Sick

When you are experiencing symptoms of cold or flu, should you continue running as normal, cut back your training, or stop running entirely? It all depends on the types and severity of your symptoms.

Most experts agree that it is okay to continue exercising as normal when you have a mild or moderate head cold, with symptoms such as sinus pressure, runny nose, cough, and sore throat. A cold that has moved into your chest, with symptoms such as chest congestion and tightness, is more likely to negatively affect your running—and if it negatively affects your running, then your running may negatively affect it. Listen to your body and your common sense in such cases. If you are able to run more or less as comfortably as usual despite your symptoms, and if running does not worsen your symptoms, go for it. Otherwise, let discretion be the better part of valor and take a day off.

When you have a stomach flu, with symptoms such as nausea, vomiting, fever, diarrhea, and body aches, you probably won't feel

Running and the Big C

Cold and flu are not the only illnesses that running wards off. A running-strengthened immune system reduces the likelihood that a variety of other diseases, including many types of cancer, will take hold in your body. For example, a large Swedish study found that men who walked or cycled for at least 30 minutes a day had a 34 percent lower risk of dying of cancer compared with couch potatoes.

Cancer starts when a genetic error occurs in the process of cellular duplication. Cells continuously reproduce in your body by making exact copies of themselves—except that the copies aren't always exact. One or more accidental substitutions of genetic material in the duplication process results in the birth of a mutated cell that is not able to function properly.

Your immune system has the job of singling out and destroying such mutant cells, and most of the time it does. But some survive, and on very rare occasions those that survive are capable of dividing and spreading out of control. The out-of-control growth and spread of mutant cells is the essence of cancer, although each of the hundreds of different types of cancer is a little different from all the others.

The first line of defense against cancer is the body's antioxidant defense system, which is not technically a part of the immune system but probably should be considered a part of it. Free radicals are often the cause of the DNA damage that creates cancer cells. As we saw in the previous chapter, antioxidants are able to neutralize free radicals, and running bolsters the body's antioxidant capacity.

Exercise is also believed to reduce cancer risk by other mechanisms. For example, high insulin levels are associated with increased risk of cancer, and exercise reduces insulin levels. Undoubtedly there are other mechanisms by which exercise combats cancer that have not yet been discovered. Fortunately, you don't have to wait for these mechanisms to be discovered to enjoy the cancer-quashing benefits of being a runner.

Even when it fails to prevent cancer from emerging in your body, exercise helps to slow, halt, and even reverse its growth and spread. Regular exercisers have a much greater chance of surviving many types of cancer than non-exercisers. What's more, cancer is significantly less likely to return in cancer survivors who exercise.

like running, and you definitely shouldn't do so. Even if you are able to log a few miles in such a condition, each one of those miles will probably add a day to your battle with the viral invader.

Also consider your training workload when trying to decide how to respond to symptoms of illness. If you train moderately, then it is unlikely that your training is suppressing your immune system and thereby possibly making it harder for you to beat the virus. So if you feel up to running, you might as well run. But if you're in very heavy training, it might be best to cut back your training, even if you're feeling okay. This will give your immune system a quick boost so it can beat the virus, preventing it from lingering as a nuisance, perhaps affecting your training for many weeks.

This recommendation receives support from the results of a 2002 study by Ola Ronsen of the Norwegian Olympic Training Center. On two different occasions, Ronsen measured various markers of immune system activity in endurance athletes after they completed a pair of workouts on a single day. On one occasion, they rested for 3 hours between workouts, and on the second occasion, they rested for 6 hours. Guess what? There was a significantly greater increase in stress hormones that compromise immune function and reduced levels of neutrophils and lymphocytes in the short-rest trial than in the longer-rest trial.

These findings suggest that an endurance athlete who's already sick will probably get well quicker if he or she takes measures to train in a more rested state, either by reducing the frequency of workouts or by making them less challenging.

Remember the story about Dathan Ritzenhein at the beginning of this chapter? It is possible that the lingering case of walking pneumonia that he took to the 2006 U.S. National Cross-Country Championships would have been nothing more than a five-day cold in another runner who was logging a fraction of the 100 miles a week that Ritzenhein ran—and that it would have been nothing more for Ritzenhein, as well, if he had cut back to 50 miles for one week as soon as it hit him. We're accustomed to thinking of high-mileage runners as hardier than their lower-mileage counterparts; in relation to cold and flu, they are in fact more fragile and must therefore sharply reduce their training in response to illnesses that 30-miles-a-week runners can train right through.

Nutrition and the Immune System

Like every other system of the human body, the immune system depends on nutrition to function properly. Much is made about how specific individual nutrients play vital roles in immune function. For example, several years ago there was a sudden explosion of "immune-boosting" supplements containing the mineral zinc, because scientists had discovered that zinc is essential to the function of the cytokines, enzymes, and hormones of the immune system. But while it is true that zinc is an especially important nutrient for immune function, it is also true that virtually any nutrient deficiency will have a negative impact on the immune system. The reductionist mentality that pervades so much of nutrition science, especially its popular interpretation, encourages us to compartmentalize immune system nutrition. We eat right for general health and then eat specific foods and take specific supplements to support our immune systems—in fact there is no legitimate distinction to be made between eating right for general health and eating to support our immune systems.

For example, protein is seldom mentioned in discussions of nutrients that are especially important for immune function, yet protein deficiency does indeed weaken the immune system. So do carbohydrate deficiency, fat deficiency, and inadequate intake of a long list of essential vitamins and minerals, while abundant consumption of technically non-essential phytonutrients contained in fruits and vegetables makes a normal immune system even stronger. So there's no point in following a special diet that is designed specifically to support your immune system. If you're already maintaining a balanced diet based on natural foods with fruits and vegetables at the base of the "pyramid," perhaps mainly for the sake of staying lean and running well, then you are already following the best possible diet for immune support.

But what about the unique immune system challenges that hard-training runners face and the supplements that are purported to address these challenges? Are they of benefit? The short answer is no. While we won't go so far as to say that all such supplements are useless for every runner, the best available research indicates that most of them have nothing to offer most runners.

The amino acid glutamine is among the nutrients most commonly taken by runners for immune support. Glutamine is used at a very high rate during exercise. It is sent from the muscles to the liver and converted to glucose, which is then sent back to the muscles to provide energy. Plasma glutamine levels drop dramatically (45 percent in one study) during prolonged exercise and remain low for some time afterward. This was believed to leave the body more susceptible to bacterial and viral infections, because glutamine is an important fuel for the immune system. Some early studies appeared to show that taking supplemental glutamine after exercise decreased exercise-induced immunosuppression and reduced the risk of infection. However, in a recent review of the scientific literature, Michael Gleeson of England's Loughborough University reported, "Several recent glutamine feeding intervention studies indicate that although the plasma glutamine concentration can be kept constant during and after prolonged strenuous exercise, the glutamine supplementation does not prevent the post-exercise changes in several aspects of immune function."

Zinc is contained in sweat, so there is some cause to speculate that runners might need to take supplemental zinc to maintain normal zinc levels and immune function. However, studies have shown that zinc levels are typically normal in nonvegetarian athletes even without supplementation and that zinc supplementation does not reduce the incidence of upper respiratory tract infection in individuals with normal zinc levels. That said, because red meat is by far the best food source of zinc, runners who eat little or no red meat should take a multivitamin-multimineral supplement that contains zinc.

Magnesium is another mineral that is vital to immune function and lost in sweat. Based on these facts, Portuguese researchers recently raised the possibility that magnesium depletion could account for a portion of the immunosuppressive effects of strenuous exercise. If this is true, then one might encourage the use of a sports drink containing magnesium during exercise to limit magnesium depletion. But we believe that nutrient depletion of any sort is not the primary cause of the immunosuppressive effects of strenuous

training. A long, hard workout is going to suppress your immune system for a short time, no matter what sort of banquet you try to wolf down during it.

This point brings us to the most commonly prescribed measure to provide nutritional support for the immune system during exercise: carbohydrate consumption. In a number of studies, the aforementioned David Nieman has shown that consuming carbohydrate during prolonged exercise attenuates the normal effects of exercise on immune parameters. But these studies may be a classic example of how science sometimes produces misleading conclusions as a consequence of creating an artificial reality in its efforts to simplify things. The problem is that in Nieman's studies, subjects were required to fast before their test workouts, so that they started them in an artificially carbohydrate-depleted state. But in a recent study in which subjects were allowed to eat a normal breakfast before their test workout, the beneficial effect of carbohydrate consumption during exercise disappeared, because the immune function consequences of prolonged exercise were themselves reduced.

The one conclusion of Nieman's research that this new study does not contradict, however, is that carbohydrate deficiency exacerbates the effects of hard training on immune function. As we saw in Chapter 8, most runners do not consume enough carbohydrate to optimize their training and racing performance. So you can expect that by increasing your carbohydrate intake for the sake of performance, you will also reduce the immune system strain imposed by your running. If your diet is generally healthy, adding more carbohydrate to your diet is the one dietary tweak we would recommend for immune support, as well as for performance support.

[Chapter 16]

In the Long Run:
Aging and Running Performance

The world-renowned heart surgeon Dr. Christian Barnard, who performed the first successful heart transplant, was once quoted as saying that he would never run, because he believed that he had only a finite number of heartbeats; and if he increased his heart rate by training, he'd use up his allocation sooner and die younger! He was no doubt being facetious—a cardiovascular surgeon's attempt at humorously finding an excuse not to exercise, perhaps? Reading between the lines, however, his joke raises some interesting questions for runners: What if running is somehow impacting your quality of life as you age? Is there a chance that distance running for a long period (decades) has long-term implications for your health? Might we one day regret our current passion for running?

The topic of aging and running is guaranteed to be a hot one because there is very little in life that is inevitable—aging is one of them! And so as we age, we should expect to experience a decline in running performance. Many aging runners fail to acknowledge this truism, and quite literally run themselves into trouble and end up fighting a losing battle against physiology.

The legend of Milo the Greek, whom we met earlier when we illustrated the key concept of overload in training (he was the child who picked up a calf every day, until it became a bull and he became the strongest man in the world) also holds a somewhat morbid and telling lesson regarding fighting this physiological battle against aging. Milo, legend has it, began to lose his strength as he grew older. He did not want to acknowledge this, and set about proving to the world that he was indeed as strong as he'd ever been. When passing a villager splitting a stump with a wedge, Milo attempted to do the same using only his bare hands. However, he only succeeded in getting his hand stuck in the tree stump, and could not remove it. While in this compromised position, he was set upon by a pack of lions and met a rather violent end. You can see a statue of his demise at the Louvre in Paris. Call it stubbornness or pride, but the point is that there are certain physiological realities associated with aging, and your running will be affected by them. That's the bad news; the good news is that you're not powerless. As a runner, you have a position of strength regarding the impact of aging on your health, provided you are sensible in your approach to training, starting right now. So let's consider those truths and how to approach them.

The Physiological Changes Associated with Aging

Aging affects numerous physiological systems, including the neuromuscular, hormonal, respiratory, cardiovascular, and metabolic systems. Perhaps the most widely known and significant changes that occur with aging are those that affect the muscle. This is precipitated by a decline in the level of the hormone testosterone. This hormone, as

any bodybuilder will tell you, is anabolic (as opposed to catabolic), meaning that it builds up tissues in response to stress, and is responsible for muscle growth and development after training. Testosterone levels peak during adolescence and early adulthood, but somewhere between 30 and 40 years of age, they begin to decline progressively.

Lean muscle mass declines, in part, due to this reduction in testosterone levels. Studies revealed a 30 percent reduction in muscle mass compared to peak muscle mass (which occurs between age 25 and 30) by age 70. This reduction involves decreases in the total number of muscle fibers as well as a decrease in the size of the fibers. Oxidative damage, described in in Chapter 14, also contributes to the reduction in muscle mass, as does a decline in the number of motor neurons that provide neural "nourishment" to the muscle fibers.

The net effect of the reduction in muscle mass is a loss of muscle strength—as much as 2 percent per year; so that by age 70, strength is reduced by up to 40 percent—though this depends on the individual and also on their activity levels. Training helps prevent these reductions, which is good news because this is the part of the equation that you can control.

As a result of reduced lean muscle mass, your body's metabolic rate declines. You'll recall from Chapter 10 that a fall in metabolic rate may tip the scale (literally and figuratively) toward weight gain, because you don't burn as much energy during the day as you did previously. Thus, it becomes more difficult to keep weight and body fat levels down as you age. Bone mineral density also decreases thanks to declining hormonal levels, and you become more susceptible to injuries. In Chapter 4 you learned that injuries happen when your training stress exceeds a "threshold for adaptation"—aging lowers this threshold, and so the injury risk increases substantially. Your body's ability to adapt to the stress of training is also reduced, and you can no longer repair damage by laying down stronger muscle fibers in response to training (see Chapter 2—DOMS).

Other hormonal changes further contribute to this adaptation barrier. The production of growth hormone decreases steadily from age 10, just after puberty, which has much the same effect as the fall in testosterone. Declining growth hormone also effects metabolism. Growth hormone has been called the "anti-aging" hormone, and is a popular choice among the Hollywood elite to retain their celebrity looks!

In women, hormonal changes are even more pronounced. Menopause and the associated hormonal changes are responsible for many effects; perhaps the most relevant for runners is decreased bone mineral density. This condition predisposes women to the development of osteopenia (a precursor to the more serious osteoporosis, which greatly increases the risk of fractures). But the excellent news is that running, because it is a weight-bearing exercise, is one of the most effective means of preventing osteoporosis. Running helps elevate bone mineral density in your younger years so that the inevitable age-induced decline does not have potentially disastrous consequences.

The number of capillaries to each muscle fiber also decreases, compromising valuable energy and oxygen delivery to muscles. Inside the muscle, proteins that are critical in assisting with metabolism are not produced in the same quantities—you therefore become less effective at producing ATP to power muscle contraction. The muscles' capacity to store and release energy changes with age—less glucose and glycogen can be stored, and the muscles become less sensitive to hormones, such as adrenaline, that normally drive metabolism. Your circulatory system also begins to show signs of aging: Your body's ability to regulate blood pressure is impaired, and your heart is less able to pump blood to your body. Your lung capacity decreases, and the ability to get valuable oxygen out of the air into the blood and to the muscles is reduced.

The net result of all these changes is that your body, which is normally a well-oiled machine, begins to resemble an assembly line which is not quite able to meet its former outputs. Every stage of the exercise process— from muscle contraction to energy formation to recovery after training—is affected.

The Impact of Aging on Performance

We all recognize that aging affects running performance. From a peak in the mid- to late-20s, most runners expect to see a decline in their running performance. Of course, some will buck this trend and do their best running in their 30s, even their 40s. Some older runners perform exceptionally well, and many will tell you that your best marathon years are your 30s. This is partly a function of the training and racing experience that is required to produce a good marathon, and also of the time it takes to move through the running ranks until you eventually commit time and effort to the marathon distance. A lot depends on the age at which you began running, how you approached it in the first few years, and of course, on your genes. There are no hard-and-fast-rules—the current world record holder is Haile Gebrselassie, age 35, while our current Olympic marathon champion is only 22 years old. The USA's brightest marathon star, Ryan Hall, is 26.

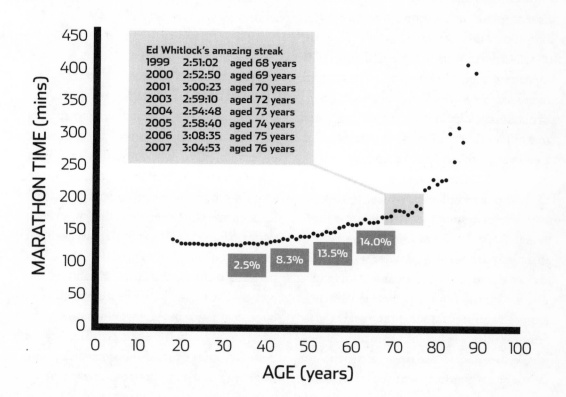

Ed Whitlock's amazing streak
Year	Time	Age
1999	2:51:02	aged 68 years
2000	2:52:50	aged 69 years
2001	3:00:23	aged 70 years
2003	2:59:10	aged 72 years
2004	2:54:48	aged 73 years
2005	2:58:40	aged 74 years
2006	3:08:35	aged 75 years
2007	3:04:53	aged 76 years

The graph on page 259 shows the World Marathon record for different ages, ranging from 18 to 90 years. There is an exponential increase in the marathon time with age—between the ages of 30 and 40, the record drops off by only 2.5 percent (this group includes the current record of 2:03:59). From 40 to 50, it falls by 8.3 percent; then by 13.5 percent from 50 to 60; and finally by 14 percent from 60 to 70. After 70, the decline is even more pronounced, probably as a result of a rapid decline in the number of runners older than 70 who participate.

If you delve into this in even greater detail, some absolutely extraordinary performances jump out. Among the most amazing of all are those of Ed Whitlock, a Canadian who holds eight age-group world records, ranging from 68 years to 76 years, including a 2:54:48 performance at age 73! Whitlock's performances are highlighted on the graph. He was the first man over 70 to run a marathon in under 3 hours; and with the exception of 2002, has set an age-group record every year since 1999.

Whitlock's story is not that unusual—though the heights he has reached are. He was an accomplished junior athlete with a mile best time of 4:31.4 at age 17 and a university 3-mile title in 14:54.4 (in 1951). He then stopped running for more than two decades, before resuming in his 40s, when he became a world champion in the over-1500 meters in the 45–49 age group. His story is fascinating for a number of reasons, but perhaps most intriguing is that his record spree began at 68, and you will not find his name on the list of marathon record-holders before this time. What is most intriguing is that there are men who were running 20 minutes faster at age 60 than Whitlock would run at 68, yet they are not featured on the list. They effectively "lost" 20 minutes in the 8-year period between age 60 and 68 years. Whitlock, on the other hand, has maintained his performances remarkably over the last 9 years, barring the odd year (2001) missed due to a knee injury. This is yet another example of the intangible quality of running longevity.

Each to His Own—The Individual Nature of Aging

One of the problems with trying to analyze the effect of aging on running performance by looking only at world records is that aging doesn't happen independently of running. In other words, using world records allows you to examine only the effect of one variable on performance. As you read this, however, your interest probably lies in how the interaction between running and aging impacts performance. The missing information in the discussion of aging and performance is often the training history. For example, if you laced your first pair of running shoes at 45, you might expect to run your best times at the age of 50. Is it valid to compare yourself at fifty to a 50-year-old running colleague who has been running for 30 years? You may be the same chronological age, but he is six times "older" than you in terms of training age. This is a relevant question.

Also, be careful not to over-interpret the world record decline, because the times in the graph are those of about 50 different individuals; and so to compare the 70-year old record to the 30-year old record is only partly useful. What you really want to do is to look at how each individual's performances change over time. Case studies of runners show that within individuals who run for more than 30 years, the decline in performance is far greater than is predicted by simply looking at world records—which stands to reason. In one example, a competitive masters runner (over 60 years old) had experienced a decline of 50 percent over a 34-year period between age 30 and age 64.

Dale Rae, an exercise physiologist at the University of Cape Town, has done some of the most detailed studies on the impact of training and aging interactions on running performance. She looked at a group of runners ranging from their 20s all the way to their 50s, who participated in 56-km ultramarathons over a period of 10 years, with the objective of teasing apart the impact of aging and cumulative training history on their performances.

Her main finding was that the age at which the first race was completed is a crucial determinant of how fast you'll eventually be able to run. Those runners who began running in their 20s were able to improve by more in the first 4 years of participation than runners who began in their 50s. This implies that chronological age is partly responsible for the capacity for performance improvement, possibly because of greater adaptability of the younger body to the training that is done in preparation for a race.

It was also shown that all the runners improved their times for 4 years and then began a progressive decline for the remaining 6 years. This means that, in general, there is a 4-year period during which you improve your performances before they decline—your PB is more likely to come in the fourth year than any other. Note that this is a massive generalization—you may know someone (you may even *be* that someone) who achieved their PB in their twentieth year of running. This illustrates one of the key points about this discussion. We have to generalize for the sake of explanation, but emphasize that aging is so individual, so difficult to predict, that we can't design an elegant formula demonstrating how you respond over time .

Returning to Rae's work, the 20-year-olds slowed down more between their fastest race (in year 4) and their final race in the 10-year observation period than did the older groups. In other words, all the runners slowed down from 4 to 10 years, but the group that started in their 20s showed the greatest decrease. This may be a function of the starting point—they were faster to begin with. An important observation: All the groups slowed down over 10 years, which suggests that 10 years of chronological aging had little effect, but rather that "training age" (10 years in all the observed runners) was the main predictor of how performance would change over 10 years.

At the end of the 10-year period, the 20-year olds, who were now 30, were running as fast as the 30-year olds had run in their very first race 10 years earlier. The same applied to the 30-year olds becoming 40—they were as fast in year 10 as the 40-year olds had been in year 1. This was also the case for the 40 and 50-year olds, and it is encouraging. It suggests that the act of running the race, and all the training it involved, did not accelerate a decline in performance. If that were true, we would expect the 20-year olds to get worse over 10 years, to the extent that they might be worse at 30 than a 30-year old starting their running career. This is obviously a finding specific to this study, its volunteers, and the specific race, but it gives reason for some optimism.

Too Much of a Good Thing? Can Long-Term Running Cause Long-Term Damage?

Now that we've seen examples of an age-related decline in running performance that is influenced by your starting age, but seemingly not responsible for an accelerated decline, we need to consider whether running too much or for very long might have negative health implications.

We've already described the effect of rapid, sudden increases in training volume or intensity on your body. Hans Selye's General Adaptation Principle has been discussed more than once to explain how high volume or high intensity training early on will push your body into an alarm stage from which it will never escape. Train too much early, and you're likely to break down injured and be forced to rest within weeks of starting your running program. This is rarely a crisis, but it is certainly frustrating. Although usually it takes just a week or two of rest, and then a more measured approach the second time around, the journey will begin anew, without the early interruption.

Then there is the negative effect of maintaining high-volume or high-intensity running for too long. In the Selye model, you will enter the period of exhaustion, where your body simply cannot adapt or cope with the repeated stress of running. You develop a syndrome called overtraining, which we described in the previous chapter: You are tired all the time; your performances fall away; and no matter how hard you train, you just cannot find the same enjoyment or ability in your running as you did even 1 month previously. Alternatively, your running body finally gives up on you—recurrent injuries, new injuries, chronic aches and pains eventually begin to limit your training. In either case, you have reached the stage of exhaustion, and you have to remove the stressor (training) for a while in order to recover, and then begin the process again. This too is frustrating, but not necessarily catastrophic; usually, a few weeks of rest, the right treatment for injuries, and a gradual return to training will put you back on track, and you'll hopefully remain in the Stage of Adaptation next time.

But what happens if you never recover from exhaustion? What happens if there is a point at which every runner's body decides that enough is enough and the marvelous adaptations to training we've described in this book no longer occur? That's the big mystery surrounding running and aging, and it introduces us to a condition that has been described as an *acquired intolerance to training*. This represents the final point of exhaustion, and there is obviously good reason to understand why it may occur.

When Adaptation Fails: Premature Aging or a More Serious Condition?

To understand the nature of adaptation failure, we return to Hans Selye's General Adaptation Principle, which has become something of an anchor point throughout this book. The diagram on page 264 summarizes the three phases in the stress response model, and summarizes very briefly some of the physiological adaptations that occur in the Alarm and Adaptation. Our concern is whether these adaptations ever fail, moving us from the Adaptation Stage into Exhaustion. It is important to understand how these adaptations change over time, so that we can appreciate why they may fail to continue adapting. This is also a concise summary of what we've described in previous chapters.

In the Alarm stage, acute responses to exercise occur—they happen during and immediately (up to a few hours) after finishing exercise. In this stage, the biggest risk is an acute injury—a torn muscle, tendon strain, or ligament damage.

In the Stage of Adaptation, the medium-term adaptations occur. These include changes in all the systems—heart, lungs, muscles, brain, metabolic. They are the adaptations that allow you to store more energy, use that energy with greater efficiency, keep your body temperature lower, activate muscles more effectively, and maintain adequate delivery of oxygen and energy to the muscles. The risk here is that the training is too hard, or too long, preventing sufficient adaptation and resulting either in an overuse injury or the early stages of overtraining syndrome. Both are immediately manageable through rest and treatment for injuries, which is usually enough to allow you to resume exercise a few

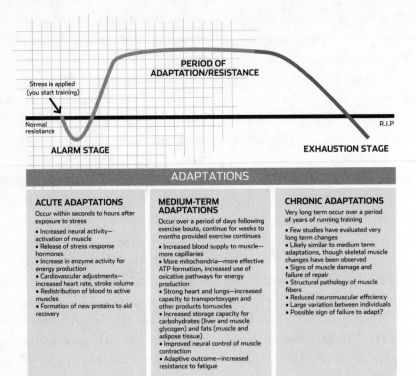

PERIOD OF ADAPTATION/RESISTANCE

Stress is applied
(you start training)

Normal
resistance

R.I.P

ALARM STAGE

EXHAUSTION STAGE

ADAPTATIONS

ACUTE ADAPTATIONS

Occur within seconds to hours after exposure to stress

• Increased neural activity—activation of muscle
• Release of stress response hormones
• Increase in enzyme activity for energy production
• Cardiovascular adjustments—increased heart rate, stroke volume
• Redistribution of blood to active muscles
• Formation of new proteins to aid recovery

MEDIUM-TERM ADAPTATIONS

Occur over a period of days following exercise bouts, continue for weeks to months provided exercise continues

• Increased blood supply to muscle—more capillaries
• More mitochondria—more effective ATP formation, increased use of oxicative pathways for energy production
• Strong heart and lungs—increased capacity to transportoxygen and other products tomuscles
• Increased storage capacity for carbohydrates (liver and muscle glycogen) and fats (muscle and adipose tissue)
• Improved neural control of muscle contraction
• Adaptive outcome—increased resistance to fatigue

CHRONIC ADAPTATIONS

Very long term occur over a period of years of running training

• Few studies have evaluated very long term changes
• Likely similar to medium term adaptations, though skeletal muscle changes have been observed
• Signs of muscle damage and failure of repair
• Structural pathology of muscle fibers
• Reduced neuromuscular efficiency
• Large variation between individuals
• Possible sign of failure to adapt?

Three phases in stress response

weeks later—but only if you obey your body early.

Next come the chronic adaptations, and this is where things get interesting—and speculative—admittedly. There are only a few studies on the very long-term adaptations of runners to many years of distance running; so much is conjecture. However, these chronic adaptations occur during the Stage of Adaptation, but there is some evidence that they may be associated with pathology that could, in theory, move some runners into a stage of Failure to Adapt and Exhaustion.

For example, one study looked at veteran runners just before a marathon, when they were supposedly in a rested state. It found that the runners' muscles displayed many of the signs of extensive muscle damage: knots, disoriented myofibrils, and the presence of some of the inflammatory cells we mentioned previously. Either the runners were not rested and had trained hard just before their marathon (unlikely), or there is some degree of muscle damage in chronically trained runners. This was supported by another study, which found many of the same signs of muscle pathology in younger runners (30 years old) who were well rested. It was concluded that repeated injury and repair caused muscle changes that were pathological for the age of the runners.

Neither of these two studies is particularly encouraging. There is, as usual, a large variation between individuals; but there is enough evidence to suggest that perhaps long-term exposure to running training causes some kind of maladaptation, which has even been described as "premature aging" of the muscle. In other words, does running age your muscles? And more worrysome, what happens next?

Intolerance to Endurance Exercise: A Common Path or a Rare Pathology?

There's no reason to be alarmed, so let's set your mind at ease upfront. These "chronic" adaptations, which have been described as pathology, are still so poorly understood that we cannot make any definitive conclusions just yet. We simply do not know whether they predict any more serious developments later in life. They are, of course, also outweighed by the many positive adaptations that runners enjoy—reduced risk of disease, reduced weight, fitness, and increased life expectancy—pretty strong incentives to run.

However, it's worth considering that some runners, for reasons that are still unknown, sometimes slip into a state during which they simply stop adapting to training.

Consider the following case study. A 64-year old runner kept meticulous training logs. (Runners can be quite particular about the details of training.) He covered 95,677 miles in training and 10,320 miles in races over 47 years. This included 90 ultramarathons and 122 marathons—88 completed in sub-3 hours. Quite a remarkable running CV. However, at the age of 64, the runner was unable to continue running. He could not sustain even a normal training load, and his performances fell away dramatically—far more steeply than would be expected for his age. He simply could not continue to adapt to the stress of running training: He had entered into the Exhaustion stage, 47 years after starting out on a very serious training regimen, and without any known cause.

There are other runners like this—some are even younger than our 64-year-old case. They were first identified by Professor Wayne Derman, of the University of Cape Town, who described a group of runners who had pronounced exercise-associated fatigue and intolerance to training. This particular group all had myopathy (pathology of their muscles) which was similar to the chronic adaptations outlined previously. So Derman named the condition FAMS, Fatigued Athlete Myopathic Syndrome. However, as more of these athletes were identified, the name was changed to ATI, for Acquired Training Intolerance, because there did not seem to be a consistent set of muscle pathologies in all the cases.

What do we know about this mystery syndrome, ATI? All of the athletes have a history of high training volume, and then experience a sudden and unexplained failure to perform—what were previously easy mid-week recovery runs became impossible to finish at half their normal pace. Tests are negative for many typical fatigue conditions, such as classic chronic fatigue syndrome and any other metabolic or neuromuscular disorders. They experience DOMS for no apparent reason, sudden muscle cramps and very tender muscles, despite training that is often less than 50 percent of what they are accustomed to. Examining their muscles through a microscope reveals a similar picture to what is seen in athletes with DOMS, suggesting that their muscles are being repaired from some damage, despite the fact that many times they are rested and have not been training. This is not a consistent finding, however, and does not suggest that running damages muscles.

Dale Rae was fascinated by the study of these runners, and found an immense challenge in trying to characterize them. Her PhD thesis was the equivalent of an exercise science episode of *CSI*, because she had to study each of these cases and then try to pick out common elements in their history, their symptoms, and their physiology. These common threads then had to be woven into a likely explanation of how the condition developed. Her work holds some significant lessons for us.

The condition is not directly caused by high training volumes and running training—for every runner who develops training intolerance, there are hundreds who do not. Also, the cases identified all share a history of high training volumes; but within that broad category, there are some very large differences between the runners who developed ATI. Some were in their 30s, with almost 20 years of running experience, others in their 50s with fewer than 10 years of running. Some had marathon PBs close to 2:30, while others were in the 3:30 range. Some averaged 2,500 miles a year in training, others averaged 4,800 miles per year. So the extensive training duration, and high mileage does not cause the problem by itself; it seems to require some other trigger or catalyst.

What was the trigger? It was all but impossible to establish definitively. It affects both men and women, and age is, as we've seen, not a likely factor. What Rae did find, however, is that all subjects displayed what she termed "co-stressors." For example, she found that four out of five ATI sufferers had continued high-volume training after being diagnosed with a viral infection. Four out of five had obsessive attitudes toward running, and three had underlying conditions including a metabolic disorder, neuromuscular abnormality, or an eating disorder. These co-stressors would compound the primary stressor, endurance training, pushing you toward the Exhaustion stage sooner.

What this means for you is that endurance training alone is probably not going to push you into running intolerance. However, if you possess these co-stressors, some of which you cannot control (having a virus, for example), then the imposition of running stress in addition to them might just be the push your body needs (and doesn't want) to develop some type of pathological state. Taking the pragmatic view, then, if you are struck down with a virus, or have a neuromuscular condition or any other potential stressor, you would be wise to avoid high training volumes. There are, of course, many reasons to avoid running while infected with a virus—the development of myocarditis, a potentially lethal heart condition is one of them. But according to this theory, you may run the risk of longer-term problems by asking your body to respond simultaneously to too many physiological stressors.

What to Do?
The Pragmatic Approach
to Running and Aging

Given the fact that aging will cause physiological changes that slow you down, and that there is little you can do to prevent these changes, the prognosis may seem dire. Add to this the fact that some athletes have abnormal muscle structure and "prematurely aged" muscles as a result of endurance running, and you'd be forgiven for thinking that running should not be at the top of your priority list as you age.

Well, don't despair. We have presented some harsh facts in this chapter, but certainly don't want to discourage anyone from continuing to run or taking up the sport. Think positively, and never forget that runners live longer, are less likely to have heart disease, to die suddenly from a preventable disease, to develop conditions like diabetes or hypertension, and generally report a better quality of life, and you'll realize that the incentives to run are everywhere. In addition, so little is known about the development of training intolerance that studies examining runners' muscles and finding signs of pathology may in fact be finding signs of continued adaptation—we simply don't know what these changes mean yet.

And finally, all those physiological consequence of aging—reduced lean muscle mass and strength, reduced bone mineral density, weight gain, and increased body fat—are all modifiable. You can, through running, slow down the decline in muscle mass and bone mineral density. You will, as a runner, be better able to control your weight by running regularly, and you will age far more gracefully than your non-running counterparts. That process starts today, regardless of how old you are—the more you can do to increase muscle mass, bone mass, and general health before you begin to experience the hormonally-controlled changes of aging, the better off you'll be in the long run, literally and figuratively.

The key is to be sensible, and manage your training, starting today and continuing tomorrow, so that you apply the same principles as you would for any other reasons—gradual change, listen to your body, and manage the stress carefully.

Index

Boldface page references indicate illustrations or tables. <u>Underscored</u> references indicate boxed text.

Concentric muscle contraction, 92

Consistency, role in injury prevention, 64

Contraction. *See* Muscle contraction

Cortisol, 227

Cortisone injections, for plantar fasciitis, 70

Cramp. *See* Muscle cramp

C-reactive protein, 155, <u>240</u>, 242

Creatine kinase, 36, 234–35

Cycling

    body temperature studies, 103–5

    DOMS and, 32, 34

    economy, 82

    high-intensity intervals, 174

    to increasing training volume, 173

    injury rate, 54–55

Cytokine hypothesis, 242–43

Cytokines, 36, 241, 242–43, 247

Dairy products, 156–57

Dehydration

    as cause of muscle cramps, 113–17

    drinking according to the Dehydration Myth, 106

    historical beliefs of runners, 96–97

    influence on health and body temperature, 100–102, **101**

    sports drink industry and, 95–98

    theories of, 99–100

    voluntary, 100

Delayed-onset muscle soreness (DOMS)

    adaptation, 33–34

    causes

        activities associated with, 32–33, 38–39

        lactate theory, 30–33

        type of running, 31–32, 38

    management, 41–42

    myths concerning, 30–33

    physiology

        damage repair, 35, 37

        eccentric muscle contraction, 34

        inflammatory response, 35–37

        muscle damage, 34–35, 38

    prevention, 39–41

    repeat bout effect, 37, 39

    scenarios for onset of, 28–30

    timing of occurrence, 32, 38

Depression, exercise as treatment for, 224–25

DEXA scanning, 48, <u>172</u>

Diabetes, 155, 164–65, <u>240</u>

Diet

    alcohol, 165

    caffeine, 164–65

    carbo-loading, 135–39, **150**

    fat-loading, 143–45

    food types

        beans, nuts, and seeds, 155

        dairy foods, 156–57

        fried foods, 157

        fruits and vegetables, 154

        grains, 155

        meat and fish, 156

        sweets, 157

    habitual, 131, 137

    high-carbohydrate for training, 137, **150**

    high-fat, <u>167</u>

    high-protein, 177–78

    for inflammation management, 241–42

    in-race energy replacement, 139–41, **151**

    matching calorie intake to calorie expenditure, 175–77

    Mediterranean, 241–42

    nutrient timing, 178–80

    quality, 157–64, **158**

Diet Quality Score (DQS), 157–64, **158**

Disinhibition, 123

DOMS. *See* Delayed-onset muscle soreness (DOMS)

Dopamine, 223, 225

Downhill running, DOMS and, 32, 38

DQS, 157–64, **158**

Drinks, for carbo-loading, 136, 139–41

Dual-energy X-ray absorptiometry (DEXA), 48, <u>172</u>

Dualist fallacy, 221

East African runners, running economy of, 85–86, **86**

Eccentric heel dip, 57, 60, **60**

Eccentric muscle contraction, 34, 38, 39, 91–92

Effort (force), 14

Electroencephalograph (EEG), 223

Electrolyte loss, as cause of muscle cramps, 113–20, <u>118</u>

Elevated backward lunge, 21, **21**

Endogenous supply, 139

Endorphins, <u>220</u>, 223

Endurance training

    increasing fat use as fuel, 142–43

    stress effect on muscle, **3**

Energy

    anticipatory regulation by brain, 196

    ATP, 12, 15, 129, 130, 133

    increase in efficiency of production, 15

    replacement during run, 139–41, **151**

Energy partitioning, 148–49

Energy products, carbohydrate concentration of, 140

Epinephrine, 227

Estrogen, 50, **53**

Excess postexercise oxygen consumption (EPOC), 174

Exercises

    ankle mobilization, 19, **19**

    cable external shoulder rotation, 27, **27**

    eccentric heel dip, 57, 60, **60**

    elevated backward lunge, 21, **21**

    lying draw-in with hip flexion, 24, **24**

    side-lying leg raise, 59, **59**

    scapular pushup, 26, **26**

    side bridge, 23, **23**, 58, **58**

    thoracic spine rotation, 25, **25**

    VMO dip, 20, **20**

    X-band walk, 22, **22**

Exhaustion, avoiding with change management, 6

Exhaustion stage, of stress response, **4**, 6, 264, **264**, 267

Exogenous supply, 139

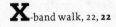